UNDERSTANDING MENTAL ILLNESS:

A Layman's Guide

UNDER-STANDING MENTAL ILLNESS:
A Layman's Guide

Nancy C. Andreasen

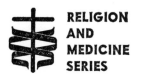

RELIGION AND MEDICINE SERIES

Glen W. Davidson, Editor

AUGSBURG PUBLISHING HOUSE
MINNEAPOLIS, MINNESOTA

UNDERSTANDING MENTAL ILLNESS

MANUFACTURED IN THE UNITED STATES OF AMERICA

To all my teachers

Contents

Foreword

Is psychiatric disorder an illness? Without reducing her answer to oversimplifications, Dr. Nancy Andreasen explains with brevity and clarity what we know today about mental illness and psychiatric care.

Many people today have sophisticated understandings of physical illness, yet when confronted by psychiatric illness, resort to misconceptions and fantasies common to the Middle Ages. Many of us have very rigid and predetermined beliefs about how our minds, and those of others around us, should function. Even if we don't understand or study formal logic, we expect behavior to reflect "common sense." While we no longer use medieval vocabulary, ascribing mental illness to the works of devils and witches, we, nevertheless, continue to make medieval assumptions about psychiatric disorders. For example, we tend to hold an individual responsible for his mental disorder: "He must have done something wrong." "She's really showing her true colors now." "He's getting what he deserves." We frequently react to psychiatric patients in ways we would not think of imposing on victims of physical disorders. Hopefully, this book will assist you to resist such tendencies and will permit you to respond with the understanding, compassion, and assistance you would give to other kinds of illness.

Illness has always been a peculiar stumbling block in Western culture. "Why illness at all?" "What does illness mean?" These are questions which recur over and over in the literature of our heritage. Both theologians and medical practitioners have debated answers to these questions. When theologians have addressed them without dialogue with medical practitioners, however, they often cast their imaginations upon speculative concerns which have had little to do with human suffering. When medical practitioners have addressed illness without dialog with theologians, they often reduced the art of therapy to the level of crass manipulation. And when discussions between theologians and medical practitioners have not included those who actually suffer illness, those discussions have often become hypothetical and abstract. Dr. Andreasen's book is one of a series designed to bridge these gaps and to speak to those who suffer illness, whether they interpret their suffering as pain of body or of soul. It is based on the latest scientific data and speaks to a particular manifestation of human suffering.

Dr. Andreasen is uniquely talented to write a book on phychiatric illness. She is a practicing psychiatrist, an author of many scientific articles, and a member of the faculty of The University of Iowa College of Medicine. She has also earned a Doctor of Philosophy degree in English literature. During her five years of teaching courses on 16th and 17th Century religious literature, she became interested in psychiatry as a way of dealing with the problems of students. Dr. Andreasen is married and the mother of two young daughters.

Glen W. Davidson, Ph.D.,
Associate Professor of
    Culture and Medicine
Southern Illinois University
    School of Medicine

1

What Psychiatric Illness Means

Now the Spirit of the Lord departed from Saul, and an evil spirit from the Lord tormented him. And Saul's servants said to him, "Behold now, an evil spirit from God is tormenting you. Let our Lord now command your servants, who are before you, to seek out a man who is skillful in playing the lyre: and when the evil spirit from God is upon you, he will play it, and you will be well."

1 SAMUEL 16:14-16

Saul was not the first victim of misunderstanding about the nature of psychiatric illness, and he was certainly not the last. The account of his problems in 1 Samuel is a moving portrayal of a gifted leader who falls prey to depression and despair in an era when such illness was interpreted by victim and bystander alike as a possession by evil spirits reflecting divine disfavor and when the only treatment available was soothing music.

You may have picked up this book because a friend or relative has experienced a psychiatric illness just as Saul did. You may have a religious background or be a religious person, and you may be feeling fear, shame, and guilt just as Saul did. Why did this happen? What did I do? Will this run in our family? Will he ever recover? How will I explain this to our friends and family? You may find it difficult to shed the ingrained feeling, enhanced by biblical passages like the one above and centuries of tradition, that mental illness is an affliction of the human spirit inflicted by an angry God. I, too, am a religious person and I believe that religion can often illuminate or help alleviate psychiatric problems, but I also believe that those who saw psychiatric illness as due to possession or witchcraft were terribly and unfortunately misguided. As a psychiatrist, I feel profound sorrow and compassion for the unfortunate individuals who for thousands of years suffered from psychiatric illness in an age less enlightened than ours. And I hope that after reading this book you will no longer feel shame, fear, or guilt; that you will become a crusader for a future age when mental illness is recognized as what it is—a disease like any other, but one which happens to affect the nervous system and, therefore, emotion and behavior rather than the heart, lungs, or kidneys.

Two hundred years ago your friend or relative might have been chained in a filthy cell for the remainder of his life, while people came to amuse themselves by observing him as if he were an animal in a zoo. Or he might have been burned at stake for being possessed by the devil. Or, if his symptoms were mild enough for him to escape these severer torments, he might simply have been an object of mockery and derision, a "bedlam beggar" taunted by small boys (or grown ones) with sticks and rocks. That is what fear, shame, and guilt about psychiatric illness have done in the past.

Even today these old ghosts haunt us. People hesitate to enter a psychiatric hospital or to encourage their loved ones to enter one. "You ought to go see a shrink" may be the final devastating insult in a bitter quarrel between two adults. We *have* improved. We don't burn schizophrenics at the stake or throw stones at the demented. But we haven't improved enough as long as people use words and phrases like "mad," "crazy," "losing his mind," or even "nervous breakdown," as long as "you need to see a psychiatrist" is a derisive taunt. And as long as some people believe that the psychiatrically ill are somehow tainted or marked for life, we still have a long way to go to conquer ignorance and fear. Hopefully, two hundred years from now both psychiatry and humanity will have progressed as far as we have in the past two hundred, and people will then look back and mourn *our* ignorance.

Your relative now sees a physician instead of being condemned for witchcraft, when he is psychiatrically disabled, and he enters a hospital rather than a prison or an "insane asylum" when he is incapacitated, because psychiatric disorders are now approached by most enlightened people through the "medical model." This in effect means that these disorders are considered as illnesses. Just as the diabetic cannot control his blood sugar by his will power but can control his illness by accepting medical treatment, so too the person with a psychiatric disorder at times behaves peculiarly for reasons he cannot understand or help but can improve with treatment. He, too, has an illness, one which affects his behavior and emotions. He deserves compassion and patience, not derision. His illness is caused by aberrations in his bodily mechanisms, as yet not fully understood, not by moral flaws or taints or a desire to be cruel and difficult. A person who suffers psychiatric disorders and his relatives have no more reason to feel guilty or ashamed than the diabetic and his relatives.

Someone may be wondering why the terms "psychiatric illness" or "psychiatric disorder" have been used here instead of "mental illness"—especially since the latter more familiar term has been used in the title of this book. "Mental illness" was chosen for the title because it is the term most people use when speaking about the subject discussed on these pages. But the word "mental" creates problems because it implies that the illness is limited to the mind. We want to avoid this implication since it cannot be substantiated. No brain abnormalities have been found on autopsy in most people suffering from psychiatric illness, and rarely do abnormalities show on an electro-encephalogram (the EEG or brain wave test). No doubt at least part of the cause is due to biochemical or neurophysiological changes in the brain as yet not discovered, but the brain is an incredibly complex mechanism which acts and interacts with a variety of other bodily mechanisms including the endocrine glands and the peripheral nervous system. Since the nervous system is involved in psychiatric illness, the term "mental illness" becomes unsatisfactory because it implies an illness limited to the mind.

Further, some people take "mental illness" to mean that their brain is damaged or that there is something wrong with their mind and that they will never be able to think clearly. In fact, most psychiatric disorders manifest themselves in the emotional or behavioral spheres, while only a few significantly affect the ability to think. This is another reason why the term "mental illness" is insufficient for our purposes.

Some readers may be wondering what psychiatric illness means in another sense. They may be wondering how one distinguishes between illness and normality in a complex area such as human behavior. Normality is itself a difficult concept. It may represent the average, what the majority of people do. Yet, a man like Einstein was far from average, perhaps even a bit odd, but could in no sense be considered psychiatrically ill. His very superiority made him in a sense abnormal, but his abnormality was desirable. Another sense of the word "normality" is that normality is an ideal. The "normal" person is one who functions to the fullest limits of his capacity. Using normality in this sense is also a bit risky, however, for few of us are able to fulfill all our intellectual and emotional capacities at all times. Psychiatrists tend to think of normality and illness in terms of ability or inability to function within the daily demands of life. Freud had perhaps the most sensible definition of what constitutes psychological health—*lieben und arbeiten,* "to love and to work." Although a person may be extremely bright or somewhat below normal in intelligence, although he may be gregarious and outgoing with many friends or somewhat shy and a loner, although he may live a conventional middle-class life or be somewhat bohemian and unconventional, he has achieved psychological health if he has learned to love some other human being and to work productively in some way which he finds personally satisfying. When a person is unable or becomes unable to function at a level commensurate with his intellectual abilities in interpersonal relations or in work, then he might be considered to have some form of psychiatric illness.

In the pages which follow, a variety of psychiatric illnesses will be described. Chapter 2 will serve as a brief introduction to psychiatric terminology and symptomatology. A word of caution should be heeded concerning that chapter. When people read about psychiatric symptoms, they inevitably tend to apply them to themselves and to think that because they occasionally have a few symptoms in a mild form, they must have the illness described. The above definition of normality in terms of capacity to function should be kept in mind. Even if you have an occasional symptom, you probably do not have or have not had the illness described unless it has affected your capacity to love and to work for several weeks or more.

2

Types of Psychiatric Illness

O the mind, mind has mountains;
cliffs of fall
Frightful, sheer,
no-man-fathomed.
Hold them cheap
May who ne'er hung there.

POEMS, GERARD MANLEY HOPKINS

Information about the types of psychiatric illness has been kept in a closet, hidden away like a frightening skeleton, for too long. Intelligent people who are familiar with the symptoms of diabetes mellitus or multiple sclerosis usually do not have an equal understanding of psychiatric disorders such as schizophrenia or even anxiety neurosis. In part, this is due to the nature of the history of psychiatry, a relatively young field in medicine. When Freud was a medical student or an apprentice neurologist-psychiatrist, the various psychiatric illnesses had not been well differentiated from one another. Our diagnoses still lack some precision today, but, nevertheless, a number of discrete illnesses have been delineated, and the layman, particularly someone who must deal with mental illness in a family member, will usually benefit from knowing psychiatric terminology.

Doctors are sometimes hesitant to give out information

concerning a diagnosis to patients or family members. If the doctor is asked directly and avoids giving a specific answer, you are certainly entitled to inquire further as to why he is hesitant. But if he persists in hesitating, he has probably made a decision that it would be contrary to the patient's welfare for him or his family member to know the diagnosis. Even if he will not give a specific diagnosis, he will probably be willing to talk openly concerning course and outcome of the illness involved. In some cases, too, doctors are hesitant to give a specific diagnosis because they are not certain as to which diagnosis is appropriate and they feel it would worry the patient or his family unduly. Neurologists who suspect multiple sclerosis are also usually hesitant to make a definite diagnosis before they are certain, as are surgeons who suspect cancer, or pediatricians who suspect mental retardation. If you have a fearful fantasy that you or a relative may have a specific illness, do bring it up and discuss it with your doctor, for usually people suspect that the illness they have is much worse than it actually is.

This chapter is designed as a brief introduction to psychiatric terminology. In the following pages, the major psychiatric illnesses that afflict humanity are described briefly. In general, the descriptions tend to follow the diagnostic terminology agreed on by the American Psychiatric Association, the professional group to which most American psychiatrists belong.

Schizophrenia

Schizophrenia is the most serious and crippling of all psychiatric illnesses. Some individuals with schizophrenia are fortunate and experience episodes of being ill which last for several months and then go into partial remission, usually with the help of medications. Some have a single episode which clears completely without leaving any deficit. Current thinking in psychiatry, however, is tending to suggest that illnesses which remit fully may not be true schizophrenia, although this is a matter of some debate. Most people who suffer from schizophrenia have a chronic illness and show at least some of its symptoms throughout most of their lives. Unfortunately, in spite of its seriousness, schizophrenia is not uncommon. One in a hundred individuals suffers from schizophrenia, and its distribution appears to be the same worldwide.

The word "schizophrenia" is of Greek origin and literally translates "split mind." Popularly, this has been taken to refer to a "split personality." The movie "The Three Faces of Eve" is believed by many people to represent what schizophrenia is like. Most schizophrenics in fact do not have split personalities at all. The Dr. Jekyll and Mr. Hyde personality change is not in any sense characteristic of schizophrenia. The name was coined in the 19th century by a Swiss psychiatrist named Bleuler, a contemporary of Sigmund Freud, who together with Freud is one of the founding fathers of modern psychiatry, although he has received much less recognition than his Austrian colleague by the general public. Bleuler coined the term in an attempt to describe the schizophrenic's characteristic "splitting of the fabric of his thoughts," to quote Bleuler himself. A typical schizophrenic usually displays a remarkable lack of connection between his thoughts and feelings.

Schizophrenia usually begins in a young person, typically during late adolescence, but it may also occur without prior symptoms in middle-aged adults. Its onset may be acute and sudden or slow and chronic. Individuals who follow a chronic course usually have a basically shy personality and are described as having been loners with few friends during childhood and particularly during their teenage years. These patients are usually described by relatives as becoming steadily more withdrawn, slowly losing interest in things they used to enjoy, and cutting down their already limited social contact to none at all. Sometimes such patients are brought in to see a psychiatrist because relatives have noticed that they do practically nothing but sit in their rooms and stare at the walls all day long, perhaps occasionally muttering to themselves. They may also become uninterested in personal hygiene and careless about their personal appearance.

Patients who have an acute onset more typically have outgoing personalities before the beginning of their illness. Like the patients with a more chronic course, they may become withdrawn, but they may also be quite anxious and agitated with strange or bizarre behavior. One young man who developed acute schizophrenia was a B student in college with a number of friends when he suddenly became ill. He began to believe that people were intentionally tormenting him, became very anxious and hostile, and indulged in magical rituals to protect himself, such as painting his shoes different colors and wearing three layers of clothing. He improved markedly after about one month of treatment.

The typical symptoms of schizophrenia may be divided into those which characterize the patient's emotional life, his thinking, and his social adjustment. The emotional symptoms are especially striking. Often the schizophrenic's emotional responses are quite inappropriate. For example, he may giggle in a foolish manner when talking about the death of a loved one. Psychiatrists call this "inappropriate affect" (affect being synonymous with emotion) and consider it a distinctive characteristic of schizophrenia. Alternately the emotions may simply be dulled rather than inappropriate. Psychiatrists call this "flattening of affect." A schizophrenic may show little or no emotion when talking about subjects which for most people would be emotion-laden. For example, he may speak calmly and matter-of-factly about the death of a loved one and exhibit no grief or sense of loss. Patients who exhibit this dulling of emotion seem to have lost the sparks of feeling that most of us have.

A second typical symptom of schizophrenia is disturbance of thinking. This, too, may take one of several forms. Sometimes schizophrenics have hallucinations. Typically the hallucinations take the form of voices, which may call them names or predict that something dreadful is going to happen. Other schizophrenics may have delusions, which are fixed false beliefs that they continue to hold persistently in the face of contradictory evidence. A schizophrenic may believe, for example, that someone is poisoning his food, controlling his body with electricity or radioactivity, or surreptitiously writing about him in newspapers. Sometimes the disturbance of thinking is not this clearly bizarre or flagrant. The schizophrenic's thought may simply seem disjointed: he jumps from one idea to another while talking without apparent connection. Observers will simply note that sometimes he does not "make sense." Sometimes schizophrenics exhibit a symptom known as "blocking." They will talk quite fluently and then stop and stare blankly, as if they had somehow lost their train of thought. These symptoms represent the "splitting of the fabric of thought" that Bleuler thought most characteristic and used to give schizophrenia its name.

A third way schizophrenics exhibit symptoms is in their social behavior. They usually have few friends and little interest in making contacts with other people. Often they are quite fearful of other people, especially members of the opposite sex. They rarely date and usually do not marry if their symptoms begin during adolescence. They have difficulty holding jobs because of their loss of interest in most things and their inability to persist in a task. They tend to show poor judgment about practical matters. Directions tend to be taken quite concretely and literally. One young man lost a job with a lumberyard, for example, when he was told to deliver an order rapidly and transported an uncovered load of valuable lumber through a rain storm so that it arrived at its destination quickly but also totally ruined. A young woman, when asked by her therapist to write down a recipe for hamburgers, wrote: "Get out a frying pan. Put the frying pan on the stove, turn on the stove. Get out the hamburger. Take off the wrapper . . . " This simple list of tasks persisted at length because she did not seem to have enough judgment to distinguish between what was important and what was simply to be taken for granted.

Some schizophrenics also exhibit paranoia. Paranoid individuals tend to be suspicious, aloof, withdrawn, hostile, and to consider themselves superior to others. They usually have a well-developed delusional system. Typically they believe that there is some complex plot going on propagated by some important agency such as the Federal Government or the FBI, which has a goal of somehow injuring or destroying them. Paranoids tend to have better judgment than other schizophrenics. Often they learn to avoid talking about their delusions and may appear normal most of the time. Usually the paranoid is dependable and has a good work history, but simply seems a little unusual and a bit of a loner.

Affective Disorder

Affective disorder is a form of psychiatric illness in which symptoms are limited primarily to the patient's mood or emotional states. Mania and depression are the two major forms of affective disorder, and these sometimes occur in alternation in the type of patient known as the manic-depressive. Patients who exhibit both mania and depression are called bipolar, while those who show depression only are unipolar.

Affective disorder is even more common than schizophrenia. Approximately two individuals out of a hundred have severe symptoms of affective disorder at some time in their lives. If milder depressions are also included, the prevalence may be as high as eight out of every hundred people. While it should be taken seriously, affective disorder is basically a less serious illness than schizophrenia. People who suffer from this illness may have many episodes of mania and depression throughout their lives or they may have only one attack. In either case, they are typically well between episodes and able to lead quite normal lives. Many famous and successful people have suffered from affective disorder, including Abraham Lincoln, Woodrow Wilson, and Samuel Johnson.

Everyone experiences mood swings from time to time. Duration and severity of symptoms distinguish a significant psychiatric illness from a simple downward mood swing. Symptoms of depression include loss of appetite, weight loss, loss of interest, chronic fatigue, decreased sex drive, diminished energy, difficulty falling asleep or early morning awakening, guilt feelings, feelings of worthlessness, and hopelessness about the future. Psychiatrists usually consider an individual who describes himself as feeling blue or depressed and admits to four or five of these symptoms for more than three to four weeks as suffering from depression. These symptoms also occur in a person suffering grief from loss of a loved one, but in this situation they are considered to represent a "normal grief reaction" rather than depression. The suffering of a depressed person is usually intense and his misery is so severe that often he contemplates suicide. Suicidal thoughts or threats in a depressed person should never be taken lightly, for most suicides occur in individuals suffering from depression. If untreated, depressive symptoms may last from several months to as much as a year, but even if untreated the depression usually goes slowly away and the individual is able to return to normal functioning. Occasionally a depressed person may feel that he is being persecuted or hear accusatory voices, but ordinarily bizarre or unusual thinking is rare in depression, and the depressed person seems quite normal except for his extreme sadness.

Depression may occur at any age. Perhaps the most typical ages for depression are in the late twenties for women and the mid-forties for men. Sometimes childbirth precipitates depression in women. Sometimes the first depression occurs in the sixties. Depression which occurs in later years (called "involutional depression" by psychiatrists) is the most difficult to treat. People suffering from involutional depression may be particularly agitated—pacing, wringing their hands, and complaining of strange and unusual pains in their body —or they may become extremely withdrawn and apathetic, refusing to eat or care for themselves in other simple ways.

At the opposite pole from depression is a condition known as mania. Some people who suffer from affective disorder experience depression only, while in others episodes of depression alternate with episodes of mania. Depression alone is quite common, but mania alone is very rare. In either case people who suffer from affective disorder have an episodic illness and are normal between episodes, although sometimes they may seem a bit more moody than the average individual.

A person in the midst of a manic attack has an exaggeration of many traits which are often considered desirable. An attack usually comes on suddenly. Uncle Bill, normally a competent, friendly, and easy-going man, will suddenly display enormous amounts of energy. He will stay up very late at night working on a project and waken refreshed at 5:00 A.M. after retiring at 1:00 A.M., getting by with little sleep without apparent fatigue. He may be too busy to have any interest in food, but he also may notice a sudden increase in appetite and eat voraciously. In spite of his furious energy, which may be directed into either a constructive or a grandiose project, his sex drive is also heightened and he may wish to have intercourse once or twice a day instead of his usual once or twice a week. When he becomes manic, Uncle Bill will become unusually jolly and seem quite euphoric. He will talk more than usual, speak very rapidly, and jump from one idea to another. His jolliness will disappear quite quickly if his plans or desires are blocked, however, and he then may become irritable, hostile, and disagreeable.

Most of the traits just described seem relatively harmless,

and indeed a typical manic feels that he is on top of the world. It can be very difficult to persuade Uncle Bill that he has a psychiatric illness. Unfortunately, however, a person in the midst of a manic attack tends to have very poor judgment. For example, one manic suffering from his first episode had been a successful real estate dealer and insurance salesman in a small midwestern city. When he became manic he decided to expand the business to Hawaii. He purchased a plane, hired four pilots to fly it, took all his employees with him to explore the area, wrote a series of bad checks and ended up deeply in debt. Early recognition of his symptoms of mania and prompt treatment might have averted this disaster. Although he had no insight at the time of his illness, when asked afterwards if he really needed four pilots, he replied, "Heavens no, I didn't need any pilots. I didn't even need a plane." Other manics may become grandiose with religious delusions. One patient, for example, felt that he was in direct communication with God and he would carry on conversations with him intermittently while also talking with his psychiatrist. He was admitted to the hospital at his wife's request because God had told him to take a plane to Miami, where he would meet Jackie Kennedy and be crowned the King of Nations while she would be his Queen of Nations.

Mania may seem normal in mild forms, and a person who is simply good natured and has large amounts of energy would not be considered manic. Poor judgment and impaired ability to function in normal life distinguish the manic from the energetic person without psychiatric illness. Mania should be considered a serious illness, but usually it responds quite well to treatment. The use of lithium carbonate, a simple alkali metal salt similar in chemical structure to ordinary table salt, has been a recent significant breakthrough in the treatment of mania. Prior to the development of modern drug therapy, mania could be a life-threatening illness, since manics would sometimes die from starvation or exhaustion.

Organic Brain Syndrome

As the name implies, an organic brain syndrome occurs when brain function is impaired by some type of physical insult. The term "organic" means that the cause of this type of disorder is physical rather than emotional. Intoxication with alcohol or drugs, personality changes secondary to brain tumor, or the impaired intellectual functioning often associated with old age are all examples of organic brain syndrome. Organic brain syndromes are usually divided into two groups, acute and chronic, because they are quite different in cause and outcome, and sometimes in symptoms as well.

An acute brain syndrome usually comes on suddenly. Some people experience their first example of an organic brain syndrome when they become seriously ill. A person who has a high fever with a serious infectious illness such as pneumonia, who has experienced a sudden debilitating illness such as a heart attack, or has suffered a massive injury such as a severe burn will often develop delirium. Symptoms of delirium are familiar to parents in a mild form if they have ever had a child who has been quite ill with a high fever. An older person who is delirious begins to behave in puzzling ways. He is not himself, he becomes confused, and sometimes he doesn't know where he is or perhaps even who he is. He may shout, become violent, and swear. Alternately he may become stuporous and lethargic. From time to time he will seem to recover from this delirium, become friendly and cooperative, recognize relatives, converse normally, seem like himself again, only to relapse into delirium much to the despair of his loved ones. The first frightening thought that comes to them is, "He's losing his mind and he'll never be the same again."

It is important that the relatives of a person with an acute organic brain syndrome realize that this state is almost always reversible. Its cure is to cure the original illness. When the high fever drops, the heart muscle functions in a more normal fashion, or the burns heal, the delirium also disappears and the patient completely recovers his normal mental and emotional functioning. It is also important for people dealing with the delirious person to recognize its fluctuating nature. The patient cannot control these fluctuations, and their cause is unknown. Relatives and friends of an individual suffering from delirium should be as calm and reassuring as possible. When the patient's doctor and the hospital permit it, a single close relative, such as a wife or child, can help the delirious patient (who also recognizes part of the time that he is confused and fears that he is losing his mind) by remaining with him as much as possible so that he is continually reoriented by a familiar face. Many of the violent or frightened responses of a delirious person arise from misinterpretation of unfamiliar surroundings such as the noises of a respirator, the beeps of monitors in a coronary care unit, or the hushed voices and movements of white-clothed individuals passing by.

A chronic organic brain syndrome, unlike an acute one, usually develops slowly, so slowly that a person in continual close contact will scarcely notice the change. This form of illness is most familiar in the elderly person who is sometimes described as senile. Usually this common form occurs because blood flow (and therefore nourishment with oxygen and nutrients) to the brain has decreased through narrowing of the vessels, diminished pumping capacity of the heart, or actual occlusion of vessels leading to the brain as in a stroke. When blood flow is diminished, the brain functions much less efficiently.

As grandfather develops a mild organic brain syndrome he will show decreased memory, often forgetting where he has put his keys or pipe or that he should zip his fly. His memory for things in the distant past will be much better than his memory for recent things, and therefore the elderly individual prefers to reminisce about his childhood because that is easier for him than discussing current events. He will find it difficult to adapt to new surroundings, and he therefore may become quite unhappy, confused, or restless if he leaves the home where he has lived for 30 years and takes a plane to California to visit his grandchildren. He will have a tendency to repeat himself and may tire the impatient by telling the same stories over and over. He may become un- expectedly tearful or unexpectedly angry even though he was once a very even-tempered person. Sometimes he may have difficulty getting to sleep at night or staying asleep and may rise in the middle of the night and wander around the house not quite knowing what to do. In an elderly person decreased hearing and vision often worsen the situation. When poor hearing and sight are added to already mildly impaired brain function, he may misinterpret his surroundings or become quite suspicious. He may even accuse loved ones of plotting against him or playing tricks on him. In the most severe forms of this illness, the person may become demented. He will not know where he is, lose control of his bowels or bladder, and make inappropriate remarks.

This type of chronic organic brain syndrome is usually irreversible. It may remain mild and not particularly trou- bling to friends and relatives, or it may become steadily worse. The relatives of an elderly person with this syndrome are often presented with a challenge. The impaired memory is best handled with love and patience. Grandfather's reminisc- ences should be listened to with attention and interest even if they have been heard many times before. The elderly person with relatively severe impairment of memory, particularly if hearing and sight is decreased too, should be spared long trips to unfamiliar surroundings. Or if trips are taken, every effort should be made to surround grandfather with familiar possessions and explain the environment and events which are occuring with a running commentary in order to decrease or prevent confusion. The elderly person who is emotionally unstable should never be taken personally. Crying spells or angry outbursts by grandfather do not mean that he has sud- denly turned against his loved ones and forgotten the many

happy years they have spent together. Paranoid suspicious-
ness is particularly difficult for loved ones to accept, but this,
like the emotional instability, must be understood and ac-
cepted as due to changing brain function secondary to aging.

Sometimes the organic brain syndrome becomes so severe,
either due to marked paranoia or to dementia, that relatives
of an elderly person must consider placing him in a nursing
home or hospital. Grandfather may, for example, refuse to
eat any food prepared by family members because he suspects
they are trying to poison him to get his money; or he may be
confined to a bed, repeatedly soiling himself and the bed-
clothes and unable to recognize people who come to talk with
him. Such situations are difficult for an elderly wife or husband or for the child who assumes responsibility for their
care. Ultimately, placing such a severely handicapped elderly
person in a hospital or nursing home is an individual decision.
It must be made taking into account the welfare of everyone
involved, including not only the handicapped person, but also
the other living relatives such as the elderly wife or the children and grandchildren.

Most of the symptoms described above are characteristic
of the chronic brain syndrome which develops during the
course of old age, and they may be regarded as the natural
results of the aging process in some individuals. But a warning should be added. Symptoms similar to those described
may also occur in other illnesses. Brain tumor, excessive use
of drugs such as sleeping pills, or excessive use of alcohol by
a middle aged or elderly person may produce similar symptoms, as may a condition known as "pre-senile dementia"
which comes on in the forties or fifties. It is quite important
that any person who evidences symptoms of an organic brain
syndrome be taken to see a physician as soon as possible and
given a thorough evaluation, particularly if these symptoms
occur in the forties, fifties, or sixties. A brain tumor or drug
abuse, for example, are treatable illnesses, and the symptoms

may be completely reversed if they are noticed and treated early enough.

Neurosis

The group of illnesses called neuroses differ dramatically from those previously discussed. In the first place, schizophrenia, affective disorder, and organic brain syndrome are probably all caused by some sort of physical factor. Neurosis, on the other hand, is generally thought to be caused by psychological factors, although this has not been definitely proved. Neurotic illness is the type Freud was most interested in, most frequently treated, and wrote most of his books about. Consequently, Freudian theory pervades the way many psychiatrists conceptualize and treat neurotic illnesses. The psychological factor causing neurosis is usually considered to be some conflict, typically arising from a childhood problem which was not completely resolved. The adult with neurotic traits thus carries with him this unresolved problem, which affects the way he relates to other people in his everyday life. Unlike the illnesses previously discussed, neuroses are usually treated on an outpatient basis and do not require hospitalization unless severe. They may be handicapping but typically are not incapacitating. Further, neurosis is universal in the sense that all of us have some. Every adult human being has neurotic conflicts and neurotic methods of handling them. Most of us do not need treatment for our mild neuroses. The descriptions which follow indicate the way in which "normal" neurosis differs from that which needs treatment.

OBSESSIVE-COMPULSIVE NEUROSIS. The mildest form of obsessive-compulsive neurosis appears in the individual usually described as having a compulsive personality. This type of person is conscientious, hard-working, punctual, tidy, perfectionistic, and often quite intellectual. The housewife whose house is never messed up and who always has well-planned meals prepared promptly for breakfast, lunch or dinner is a familiar example of this type of personality. So, too, is the hard-working businessman who is a stickler for details. Usually compulsive traits work for the benefit of the individual possessing them and often for his associates, though compulsive people are sometimes difficult to be around. The tidy housewife may nag her husband and children excessively about dirtying ashtrays or messing up the house while playing, and the detail-oriented businessman may irritate his associates with complaints which seem petty.

The compulsive can be quite contemplative, worry a great deal, and have trouble making decisions. In spite of his superficial orderliness, he usually has one area of his life where he is extremely uncompulsive and messy. Psychiatrists summarize this with the saying, "Scratch a compulsive and you'll find dirty underwear." The compulsive has trouble showing, recognizing, and expressing anger. Consequently, he is unusually pleasant to have around and seems quite mild mannered. Unable to "blow his stack," he may irritate others by continually nagging or picking at them.

The compulsive personality was usually brought up by parents similar to himself. They too were conscientious and perfectionistic and encouraged the development of these traits in their offspring. Freud thought that compulsive personalities were often produced by excessively harsh toilet training, but this is probably an oversimplification. The compulsive is usually a successful person who rarely needs or seeks psychiatric treatment. This is perhaps the one form of neurosis which tends to promote successful adjustment in our achievement-oriented society. The chief hazard a compulsive faces is the development of depression when his ability to achieve his ideals is frustrated, either through personal limitations or through being blocked by some external force. For example, a compulsive individual finds it difficult to bear physical illness, because most of his life is organized around keeping busy and performing tasks. If he makes a serious error, he tends to develop guilt feelings out of proportion to the actual act. Thus on these occasions his conscientiousness and perfectionism may get in his way and he may develop a depression of sufficiently significant proportion to need psychiatric treatment.

A full-blown obsessive-compulsive neurosis differs from the compulsive personality just described by being much more severe. Instead of being simply perfectionistic, these people find their entire lives governed by obsessions and compulsions. Bill, a Ph.D. chemist, was an obsessive-compulsive neurotic who found himself in need of treatment. He possessed the typical underlying compulsive personality. He was a minister's son, strictly reared, who when only 20 married a widow several years older with a small child. After they had been married for about five years, he found himself growing gradually incapacitated by a compulsion to wash his hands repeatedly when he was under severe professional stress at work and financial stress at home. The problem was brought most sharply in focus by his compulsive need to wash his hands after playing with his stepson. He sought treatment when both the boy and the mother indicated how distressing they found this behavior. He improved after three or four months of psychotherapy, in which he explored his inability to express his feelings, his excessive conscientiousness, and his considerable (but previously unrecognized) anger toward authority figures.

A few obsessive-compulsives have a very severe form of this illness. These people are so handicapped by their obsessive thoughts and their compulsive rituals that they are literally unable to accomplish anything. They may spend hours after getting up in the morning buttoning and unbuttoning and rebuttoning their clothes in order to get it done just right. Fortunately, such severe forms of this illness are rare.

ANXIETY NEUROSIS. Anxiety neurosis too may range from mild to severe. The tense, nervous individual who is a continual worrier is the prototype of the mild form of this problem. Like the compulsive, he usually functions quite success-fully because his neurotic tensions and fear of failure drive him on to achievement. The mildly anxious individual rarely needs or seeks treatment, although he probably suffers more personal discomfort than the mildly compulsive individual, for his is a problem of irrational fear, which is subjectively unpleasant. Freud thought that the person suffering from anxiety neurosis actually experienced some overwhelmingly fearful event in childhood which he then forgot or repressed because it was so painful. Yet the memory of this fearful event lurks in his unconscious and haunts him.

The anxious individual only needs and seeks treatment when he finds his anxiety handicapping. Often the stimulus to seek treatment is an experience which psychiatrists call an "anxiety attack." This consists of a subjective experience of an irrational fear or panic, feelings of impending doom, ac-companied by physical sensations such as shortness of breath, pounding heart, sweaty palms, and queasiness in the stom-ach. These symptoms may be brought on by a realistically fear-provoking situation, such as when a student is called on in class, when a person is unable to perform satisfactorily sexually, or when a man is called on the carpet by his boss. But severe anxiety attacks frequently occur without any pre-cipitating stimulus and, therefore, are irrational in nature. Treatment usually consists of tranquilizing drugs, psycho-therapy which aims at helping the individual understand the sources of his anxiety, or a combination of both.

PHOBIC NEUROSIS. Phobic neurosis (Greek, *phobos*, or fear) is related to anxiety in that it too is based on a crippling sense of fear. In Freudian theory, phobic neurosis is caused by the same sort of primal overwhelmingly fearful experience as anxiety neurosis. Most of us have some mild phobias. Another psychiatric truism is that "every person is entitled to have one or two phobias." Some common relatively normal phobias are fear of high places, fear of being trapped in an elevator, or fear of animals such as snakes or spiders.

A phobia should only be considered troubling when it handicaps an individual's ability to function. Mr. Mason sought treatment, for example, when he found his fear of traveling too far from home kept him from enjoying forms of recreation which he valued highly. He was a successful retired businessman who enjoyed fishing and hunting. His mother died when he was only eight, and he witnessed her death. He was again orphaned at sixteen when an older sister who had been caring for him died. He worked hard, invested wisely, and eventually built up a substantial fortune. He married in his late thirties and had no children. He had an extremely close relationship with his wife and first began to experience his fear of leaving home after he retired in his early sixties. His retirement had been precipitated by having a heart attack from which he recovered fully, but which led him to the decision to spend the remainder of his life enjoying himself. As he talked more and more about his phobia, it emerged that his primary fear was of death, particularly of death while separated from his wife. He evolved the magical belief that he would not die as long as he was close enough to get back to her and have her hold his hand. In this particular case, helping him understand that his fear of dying alone probably was based on his prior abandonment by two important mother figures in his life was of little help. Neither was the Roman Catholic faith in which he had been raised. This particular case responded well to behavior therapy— simply separating him from his wife and encouraging him to travel farther and farther from home, which eventually led him to realize that nothing drastic would happen if he were in fact separated from her by long distances and long periods of time.

HYSTERIA. Hippocrates, the father of modern medicine, coined the term hysteria to describe emotional disorders which he observed primarily in women. Their primary symptom was difficulty speaking or swallowing. He hypothesized that their uterus (Greek, *hysterikos)* had been displaced and wandered up to block their throat. In fact, the disorder occurs, although more rarely, in men as well.

Hysteria sometimes appears in a milder form, usually called a personality disorder rather than a neurosis by psychiatrists. A person who has a hysterical personality is rather immature, emotionally unstable, and tends to describe his or her experience in a rather dramatic and flamboyant way. Hysterics have difficulty forming deep and lasting emotional relationships with others and place a great emphasis on appearances. They often complain of multiple physical ailments for which no cause can be found.

The disorder which Hippocrates described is the more severe form, hysterical neurosis. Psychiatrists divide this into two types, the dissociative form and the conversion form. Dissociative neurosis occurs when the person experiences a severe and sudden personality change, similar to the split personality popularized in film and fiction. The person is in a dreamlike state and performs acts he is unaware of. In the conversion form the person suddenly suffers from a dramatic physical symptom such as seizures, paralysis, inability to speak or swallow, or severe abdominal pains. The symptoms appear so severe and convincing that the disorders are often treated either medically or by surgery, but in fact on careful study no physical basis can be found.

"Anna Peterson" illustrates both the dissociative and the conversion form of this illness. She was a very attractive young woman, apparently happily married to an artist husband and the mother of three small children. Because her husband had chosen not to work for a year in order to have more time to devote to his painting, she began to work evenings as a waitress for dinner parties at the local country club. One night while serving for a poolside party she slipped, fell, and struck her head on the edge of the pool. She lost consciousness for several minutes but, although stunned thereafter for an hour or two, she seemed to have recovered fully by the next day. Several months later she began to suffer from a seizure disorder in which she would cry out and then shake with her entire body. A complete neurologic workup demonstrated no cause for the disorder and no relationship to the fall. She was placed on medication but the seizures worsened. She also began to have dissociative episodes in which she would disappear for a day or two at a time, taking the family car and suddenly coming to herself hundreds of miles from home. She began to go from neurologist to neurologist to find the cause for these ailments, and when repeatedly none could be found she was eventually hospitalized in a psychiatric institution. There hypnosis was used as a means of treatment, and eventually material was uncovered which indicated that she felt unresolved anger toward her husband for requiring her to work and raise her children, and also unresolved sexual feelings toward her father. When this material was lived through in hypnosis and brought to a conscious level afterwards, she eventually recovered fully.

Hysteria is the most dramatic of the neuroses, as the case of Anna illustrates. Freud earned his living by treating wealthy Viennese women suffering from this ailment. It was through working with them that he developed his theories of the unconscious, the "talk it through" therapy that eventually became psychoanalysis, and his theories about infantile sexuality, fixation, regression, and the Oedipus complex. Most of the women he treated described sexual feelings for their fathers and actual rape by them. Initially Freud believed these stories, but when they began to occur repeatedly his stolid middle-class temperament finally led him to doubt their truth and he recognized that in fact the stories represented wishfulfilling fantasies. For some reason such severe forms of hysteria are relatively rare today. Further, not all hysterics neatly fulfill Freud's theory that hysteria results from unresolved feelings of love toward the father.

Alcoholism and Drug Abuse

ALCOHOLISM. Alcohol is one of the world's oldest drugs. Through the centuries it has been used as a tranquilizer, an antidepressant, an anesthetic for labor pains or minor surgery, and a liquid sleeping pill. Use of alcohol is very widespread and many physicians follow St. Paul and suggest taking a little wine as a means of enhancing the appetite and calming the nerves. Conditions encompassed by the general term alcoholism range from what might be called "problem drinking" to a severe condition which involves physical dependence on alcohol and physical and mental deterioration secondary to excessive use.

When should one begin to worry that use of alcohol may be excessive? Perhaps a sensible guideline is that someone who takes more than two drinks on a daily basis is potentially headed for a problem. The individual who abstains during the week but habitually drinks himself blind on the weekends is also potentially headed for a problem.

Psychiatrists decide that the problem has become real rather than potential on the basis of a number of indicators. One of these is physical symptoms. People who use alcohol to excess often develop physical problems such as abdominal pains due to gastritis or ulcers, blackouts, delirium tremens, or cirrhosis of the liver. Perhaps the most severe complication is a condition known as Wernicke-Korsakoff syndrome in which the individual becomes uncoordinated, has paralysis of his eye muscles, suffers from poor memory, and is unable to learn new material. Another indicator that problems with alcohol are becoming severe is a variety of behavioral manifestations—missing work, becoming quarrelsome under the influence of alcohol, making suicide attempts while drinking, having marital difficulties, being arrested for drunken driving, or having a car accident while intoxicated. The third indicator is certain drinking patterns such as an inability to stop drinking once started, drinking before noon, and drinking while at work.

A person who has been drinking excessively usually develops a physical dependence on alcohol and has withdrawal symptoms when he is no longer able to drink. Symptoms of withdrawal from alcohol can be serious and life-threatening, for in addition to tremor, fever, sweating, subjective discomfort, seizures and severe changes in blood pressure may occur. For this reason a person physically dependent on alcohol should always be truthful about his alcoholic intake when placed under circumstances when he may be deprived of alcohol. For example, a businessman who drinks heavily and is admitted to the hospital for routine surgery such as hernia repair may develop symptoms of alcoholic withdrawal if he attempts to hide his dependence on it. Withdrawal symptoms can be prevented or reduced if the physician is aware of the dependence and prescribes tranquilizers.

Living with an alcoholic can be difficult and heartrending. Furthermore, alcoholism is one of the most difficult forms of psychiatric illness to treat. Nevertheless, a variety of options are open. One of these is Alcoholics Anonymous. AA stresses total abstinence and uses regular group meetings in which members provide mutual support for one another as a means of maintaining this total abstinence. AA is not helpful for everyone, however, for its evangelical emphasis on recognizing one's error and reminding oneself of it continually is distasteful to some people. But it is perhaps the single most effective means of handling alcoholism.

Another resource for the alcoholic is the general physician. He may help in the supervision of medical problems which arise secondary to alcoholism and by prescribing medications which may help control the drive to drink. Tranquilizers are often prescribed for alcoholics to substitute for the tranquilizing effects of alcohol. Antabuse (disulfiram) is a drug which alcoholics take voluntarily, knowing that if they drink within five days after they have taken an antabuse tablet they will become physically ill with extremely unpleasant symptoms. Antabuse can be helpful to highly motivated alcoholics in preventing impulsive drinking binges. Rarely, alcoholics may wish to visit psychiatrists. A psychiatrist can help an alcoholic examine his reasons for drinking, prescribe antabuse or tranquilizers like the general physician, and provide individual support and encouragement for abstinence.

DRUG ABUSE. Although more attention is focused on drug abuse among young people, drug abuse is in fact a significant problem among young and old alike. Each age group has its characteristic drugs which it abuses. Those of the young include marijuana, LSD, "uppers," and "downers." Heroin also tends to be a problem among the young rather than the old simply because heroin addicts rarely live to be old. In addition to alcohol, the drugs which older people abuse include diet pills, tranquilizers, and sleeping pills.

Many parents wonder how they can recognize signs of drug abuse in their children. Perhaps the single most suggestive sign is a dramatic personality change, especially withdrawal and loss of interest in activities previously enjoyed. A youngster using "uppers" and "downers" may have periods of excessive sleepiness and excessive energy in alternation. Marijuana users often have red watery eyes and appear mildly sedated. Very obvious signs include finding drug paraphernalia such as foul-smelling pipes or hypodermic syringes, pills of any kind, or needle tracts on the arm. A parent who notices indicators such as these should simply confront his child directly and kindly. If the suspicion of drug use turns out to be correct, then the youngster should be evaluated by a professional if his drug problem seems to be severe.

What constitutes a severe drug problem? Which drugs are dangerous? LSD is still in use, although its vogue appears to be passing as more and more people have become aware of the hazards involved in LSD use. LSD can produce acute psychotic episodes in which the user becomes panic-stricken and terrified. The death of Art Linkletter's daughter while on such a "bad trip" brought the hazards of LSD usage to widespread popular attention a few years ago. Occasionally young people who have used LSD repeatedly may also suffer from a residual state similar to schizophrenia. Generally speaking, LSD should never be used, for it cannot be predicted when an individual is going to have a bad trip. Furthermore, what is often sold as LSD may contain other dangerous substances such as strychnine.

Amphetamines or "speed" are another potentially dangerous drug, for repeated use can produce a state known as "amphetamine psychosis." The symptoms of amphetamine psychosis include difficulty sleeping, a preoccupied repetition of simple tasks, paranoid suspicion, and unexpected outbursts of anger. Clinically, amphetamine psychosis is also similar to schizophrenia.

The dangers of heroin can simply not be overestimated. The drug is so pleasurable that using it even one time may lead to addiction. Repeated heroin usage, in addition to demanding that the user pay for his habit with criminal behavior because it is so costly, also inevitably leads to physical illness such as hepatitis or other infections. Many heroin addicts die of accidental overdoses.

Marijuana, in contrast, is probably most dangerous simply because it is illegal. Chronic marijuana usage does not lead to addiction, although it may produce a mild psychological dependence. It is probably no worse in this respect than alcohol, and the physical and emotional problems associated with marijuana usage may actually be less than with alcohol. Nevertheless, laws against marijuana remain on the books at present and consequently few parents will want their children to become involved with it.

Older people can also have drug problems, although they are more prone to ignore them. Amphetamine usage is perhaps a more serious problem among middle-aged housewives than it is among young people. The older person takes amphetamines for different reasons than the young person. He usually conceives of them as diet pills rather than speed and uses them both to keep his weight down and to increase his pep and energy. Until quite recently, diet pills were abundantly available to this age group, which had the economic power to pay for them. Consequently, there has actually been more risk of dependence and amphetamine psychosis in the middle-aged than in the young.

The second group of drugs which older people abuse most commonly are barbiturates and tranquilizers. Often these are prescribed for a person who has mild anxiety and some difficulty sleeping. The sleeping pills are very helpful at first, but then a phenomenon known as tolerance begins to occur. The person's body becomes accustomed to the drug, and increasing doses are required to get the same effect. The average dose prescribed to produce sleep with a barbiturate is about 100 mg. Middle-aged people will appear in psychiatric hospitals on dosages as high as 1000 or 1500 mg., having gradually increased the dosage in order to counteract their insomnia and anxiety. Often they have gotten their pills from a variety of physicians who were not aware of the person's dependence. Signs suggestive of dependence on barbiturates or tranquilizers are slurred speech, impaired balance, staggering, falling, or car accidents.

The hazards of tranquilizers are similar to barbiturates but they are likely to be milder because these drugs are less habit-forming and tolerance is developed less quickly. As in the case of physical dependence on alcohol, sudden withdrawal from barbiturates or tranquilizers can be a serious matter, and again such physical dependence should never be hidden from a physician. Sudden withdrawal of barbiturates can produce seizures, brain damage, and acute psychosis. If the drug is withdrawn slowly, depression often follows afterwards. People who have been taking large amounts of drugs such as LSD, amphetamines, heroin, or barbiturates and tranquilizers will ordinarily require hospitalization.

Disorders in Children

THE HYPERACTIVE CHILD. The syndrome known as hyperactivity is quite common, occurring in approximately four percent of schoolage children. It is much more common in boys than girls. In the past it has been labeled with other names such as "minimal cerebral dysfunction" or "minimal brain damage." These terms are best avoided, since the causes of hyperactivity are not known definitely, and many children suffer severe assault to their self-esteem when they are made to feel that their brain is damaged by being given such labels. The syndrome of hyperactivity has no specific relationship with intelligence, and it can occur in the very bright as well as children with intelligence below normal. Hyperactive children are sometimes the product of a difficult pregnancy, a prolonged labor, or a difficult birth, and sometimes it is associated with neurological problems such as clumsiness, perceptual reversals, or left-right confusion. This has led some psychiatrists to suspect that there may in fact have been some minimal cerebral trauma, but if so it is a type of trauma which probably affects behavior rather than intellectual ability.

The classic symptoms of the hyperactive child are restlessness, excitability, distractability, and impulsivenes. In school, teachers notice that the child has difficulty sitting still for long periods of time, cannot pay attention to tedious tasks, and is prone to clown to get the attention of other children. Often children are first brought in for treatment when they enter kindergarten because their restless behavior and short attention span make them difficult to manage in the classroom situation.

Usually the child's mother has noticed long before that Johnny is difficult to manage. He gave up his nap early, usually before two years, and during his waking hours was restless, curious, and often destructive. He was difficult to get to bed at night and seemed to require very little sleep. Sometimes hyperactive children have more difficulty achieving bowel training than bladder training, and they have a tendency toward constipation. The abundance of energy and curiosity which normal children have is magnified many times in the hyperactive child, and he can move from pouring oatmeal on the floor to unraveling all the toilet paper to emptying out all the wastepaper baskets with astonishing rapidity. He shows little "common sense" and will impulsively run out in the street without looking or jump into deep water when he does not know how to swim. He tends to ignore painful stimuli, and often spankings are of little help in disciplining him and may make him worse.

When he finally does get to sleep at night, he is a restless sleeper who tosses and turns and whose bed is difficult to make in the morning because of the tangled sheets. He sweats a lot and may awaken in the middle of the night with night terrors—a state different from nightmares in which the child shouts out and appears frightened but remains in a dreamlike state and cannot recall what happened after awakening. Hyperactive children are also more likely to be sleepwalkers than other children. They often have rather poor coordination and are slower to learn to swim or ride a bike than their peers. Because of their restless and often destructive behavior, their emotionality, and their attention-seeking behavior, they often have trouble getting along with children their own age.

The treatment of hyperactivity is often double-barreled if the problem is severe. The hyperactive youngster should be evaluated by a physician who may recommend the use of cerebral stimulants such as Ritalin or Dexedrine. Paradoxically, these medications which are so stimulating to adults have a tranquilizing or sedative effect on the hyperactive youngster. They are quite effective in increasing his attention span and diminishing his distractability, and therefore they are particularly useful when he is in the classroom.

The second mode of treating hyperactive children is

through good disciplining and parenting at home. All children need firmness, consistency, and affection, but the hyperactive child needs these in more abundance than most. Because his emotional and destructive behavior tends to alienate others, the hyperactive child often suffers from a poor self-image and low self-esteem. He comes to feel that he is unpopular, a "dummy," and a "bad kid." Firm rule setting is necessary for these children, and rules should be enforced with absolute consistency. Perhaps the most effective form of punishment for a hyperactive child is isolation rather than spanking. Sending him to his room for fifteen minutes or a half hour will cut down the stimuli which have "cranked him up" and led him to misbehave, and he will usually emerge calmed down.

LEARNING DISABILITIES. Learning disabilities are often associated with hyperactivity, but either problem can also occur in isolation from the other. Learning disabilities are also not related to intelligence. By definition, a learning disability occurs when a child is more than two years behind the level appropriate to his mental age (not chronological age) in a specific subject. If Johnny has a normal IQ (a mental age of ten years when he has a chronological age of ten years) and is reading at a level appropriate to an eight year old, then he probably has a specific learning disability in reading.

Like hyperactivity, learning disabilities are more common in boys than in girls. Often they tend to run in families, suggesting that there may be a heredity factor. One often hears that grandfather never learned to read and that uncle Jim only succeeded in learning after much difficulty. Now little Johnny is coming in for an evaluation in the first grade because his teacher has noticed that at the end of the first semester he has fallen markedly behind the other children. If Johnny is indeed brought in in first grade, one should rejoice. Learning disabilities are best handled when they are caught early and appropriate teaching methods initiated before the child gets too far behind.

We still have much to learn about learning disability. The youngster who is having difficulty learning should probably be evaluated with testing of his vision and his hearing to rule out some specific physical cause. As yet we know of no way to change the defect if one is present. Instead it must be worked with and compensated for. The child will ordinarily be placed in a special program which will help him handle his specific problems. For example, he may need more drilling on fundamentals. Or he may have already developed such severe feelings of frustration and failure that he will need to be given his assignment in small "dosages" which he feels more able to handle; whereas children in a regular program may get fifty problems on one page, the child with difficulties in math may be given ten problems on five pages.

Parents can provide considerable help for the child with learning disabilities. Most importantly, they can prevent further losses of self-esteem. They should help him look for an area where he genuinely excels, such as sports or artistic skills, and then give him enthusiastic praise for his success in these areas. They can often supplement schoolwork by providing amusing ways to work on fundamentals such as phonics or mathematical facts at home. This can help the child increase his vocabulary by teaching him new words at home, improve his ability to abstract by playing games like "animal, vegetable, or mineral," or have him make up stories or describe things he sees. A child with difficulty in mathematics can be given a few addition or multiplication problems to solve at the dinner table, beginning at first with simple ones that he is able to do well. The child should be given lots of positive reinforcement in the form of praise for his success, and the problems should be gradually increased in difficulty.

What Causes Psychiatric Disorders?

Where there is much desire to learn, there of necessity will be much arguing, much writing, many opinions; but opinion in good men is but knowledge in the making.

AREOPAGITICA, JOHN MILTON

It is only natural for the person suffering from a psychiatric disorder or his relatives to ask the question "Why me?" Only one hundred years ago people would have replied to themselves that they were somehow being punished for a sin they or their forebears had committed. As we will see in the final chapter, there may be some sense in which sin and guilt do contribute to the development of illness. But ordinarily, though religion may do much to help the individual suffering from psychiatric illness, it can do little to explain its cause. Psychiatry does have a variety of theories and hypotheses concerning what causes psychiatric illness but it also has much to learn still.

The Medical Model

According to the medical model, psychiatric disorders should be considered as medical illnesses analogous to diabetes mellitus or coronary artery disease. The emphasis in this model is on carefully diagnosing each specific illness from which the patient suffers, just as an internist would carefully determine what specific illness is causing shortness of breath in the patient who comes to see him with this complaint. It is assumed that a specific cause for each specific disease will eventually be discovered, and in the meantime the search for that specific cause is aided by carefully observing the symptoms of the illness, its course, response to treatment, and the family history of the person suffering from the illness. The search for specific causes of specific illnesses has to this point focused on two areas, biochemical aspects and genetic aspects.

Much of the thrust of current psychiatric research has been directed toward finding a chemical factor which causes psychiatric illnesses. In internal medicine, for example, the diagnosis of diabetes is made through simple blood and urine tests which give a clear-cut indication of whether a person is seriously diabetic or borderline diabetic. At present, no such clear-cut and simple technique exists in psychiatry. Psychiatrists at the present time must rely on careful observation of symptoms, clinical observations, and family background in order to determine a diagnosis. The dream of most psychiatrists is to find a laboratory test which will provide an accurate diagnosis and possibly also help identify susceptible individuals, just as the glucose tolerance test does in diabetes.

Since the early days of psychiatry, specific brain abnormalities have been sought for in individuals with psychiatric disorders. But postmortem examinations of individuals suffering from psychiatric disorders disclose no such abnormalities except in individuals suffering from organic brain syndrome, alcoholism, or syphilis. The two major psychiatric illnesses, schizophrenia and affective disorder, as well as the neuroses, show no such abnormalities. Consequently, most people feel that the problem must be at a smaller, finer level, which leads them to believe that it is probably biochemical.

The search for biochemical origins of psychiatric disorders is necessarily slow. In the first place, we have come to realize that the brain, rather than the heart, is the true physical source of life, and one dare not tamper with the brain in human beings for experimental reasons. Unlike other illnesses, such as tumors, psychiatric illness is limited to human beings and animal research yields little reliable data. Furthermore, the brain is extremely complex. Even if one were able to examine blood traveling to and from the brain, techniques for which are rather hazardous and therefore constitute unethical experimentation in human beings, one might not obtain a great deal of insight in any case. For the biochemical factors producing disorders are most likely located in a particular area of the brain and measurement of blood samples would not necessarily isolate them.

For example, we now know that Parkinson's disease, a neurological disorder, is probably due to a biochemical malfunction in the area of the brain known as the substantia nigra, which is deficient in a chemical known as dopamine. But in psychiatric disorders the malfunctioning area could be in the temporal region, which controls speech and memory, in the frontal lobe which is thought to control subtle personality functions and emotions, in the hypothalmus which controls appetites and emotions, or in the "associative" regions which interconnect various parts of the brain. As yet, none of the psychiatric disorders has been specifically localized in the same manner that Parkinson's disease has been.

A number of specific hypotheses are currently being applied in the search for a biochemical factor in psychiatric disorders. One of the most popular is the "catecholamine hypothesis" for affective disorders. Catecholamines are chemical substances stored at the ends of nerve cells connecting one cell to another, known as synapses. The release of catecholamines causes a nerve impulse to be conducted from one nerve to the next; therefore, they are known as "neurotransmitters." Unusually large amounts of catecholamines have been found in the blood and urine of people suffering from mania. Decreased amounts have also been noted in people suffering from depression. Therefore, the catecholamine hypothesis suggests that mania results from a biochemical abnormality in the brain due to excessive amounts of catecholamines. This causes nerves to fire too often and too much, thereby leading to manic energy and excitement.

On the other hand, in depression a catecholamine deficit would produce a generalized depression of the central nervous system and thereby the psychological symptoms of depression such as decreased energy. The catecholamine hypothesis is at present simply a hypothesis and has not been definitely proved. It is to some extent born out by the action of antidepressant drugs, which increase amounts of catecholamines in the brain.

In the case of schizophrenia, a variety of competing theories are currently operating. Since schizophrenics often are quite agitated and excited during the early stages of their illness, catecholamines have also been suggested as a possible cause of schizophrenia. A "pink spot" has been found in the urine of acute schizophrenics and a catecholamine-like substance has been found to produce this pink spot. Taraxein (Greek, *tarassein,* meaning "to disturb") is another chemical factor which has been implicated as a cause for schizophrenia. Taraxein is a substance extracted from the blood of schizophrenics which has been claimed to produce psychotic symptoms when injected in monkeys. Yet another theory, perhaps the most promising, suggests that the biochemical abnormality in schizophrenia is a defect in the enzymatic apparatus involved in adding methyl groups to amino acids. This hypothesis has been given partial confirmation through studies of the mechanism of action of drugs such as chlorpromazine, which is quite effective in counteracting schizophrenic symptoms and also inhibits methylation. Ultimately, the defect in schizophrenia is probably due to improper activity of neurotransmitters in a specific area of the brain, probably one of those areas which controls personality or emotions, although the defect could be diffuse.

If some psychiatric disorders are due to biochemical abnormalities in the brain, then what causes these biochemical abnormalities to occur? As in the case of other medical illnesses, this more distant cause is probably due to some type of abnormal interaction between heredity and environment. That is to say, there may be a genetic factor predisposing to psychiatric disorder which is activated by some type of disturbance in the environment. For example, diabetes mellitus tends to run in families and, therefore, a genetic factor may be involved. And yet a person with a positive family history for diabetes mellitus has a greater likelihood of developing it himself if he has poor eating habits, becomes obese, or uses alcohol excessively.

Observers have long noted that psychiatric disorders, especially schizophrenia, tend to run in families. An investigator named Kallmann did one of the earliest studies in which he attempted to determine the role of heredity. Examining twins, he found that identical twins had a 58 percent concordance rate for schizophrenia. In other words, if one twin develops the illness, then the other identical twin has a 58 percent chance of also developing it eventually. Most of the remainder show some schizophrenic traits but about 10 percent are quite normal. On the other hand, non-identical twins have only a 15 percent concordance rate. Since identical twins have the same genetic material and fraternal twins do not, these data strongly suggest that the genes play a significant role in producing schizophrenia. Of course, one wonders why 10 percent of identical twins show no symptoms of schizophrenia. This clearly implies that an environmental factor, broadly defined, must also interact with the genetic factor to produce schizophrenia. This might include a variety of factors, such as intrauterine or birth trauma, upbringing, or the stresses of adult life.

Only in schizophrenia has the genetic factor been so clearly demonstrated. There are no carefully designed twin studies or adoption studies as yet for other psychiatric disorders but family studies have been done which imply familial patterns of illness in affective disorder, alcoholism, and hysteria. Since they have not separated environmental and hereditary factors in the experimental design, they at present do no more than suggest that hereditary factors may be involved.

What are the implications of these findings for the families of people suffering from psychiatric disorders? They will inevitably wonder whether they or their children will also inherit the disease from which their relatives suffer. There is, of course, some chance of this but one should not be unduly concerned. First of all, the odds are low, even in those disorders in which a genetic relationship has been "proved" by relatively pure research. Only about 15 percent of the siblings of schizophrenics develop the illness, and only about 16 percent of their children develop it. Secondly, environmental factors seem to play a significant role, even in individuals whose heredity may indicate a tendency to psychiatric illness. To some extent, environmental factors can and may be manipulated in order to prevent the development of the illness just as they can be in diabetes. Thirdly, the prognosis of psychiatric illnesses is no longer dismal, should such an illness develop. Relatively successful treatment programs have been developed for the illnesses in which hereditary factors may play a role, particularly affective disorder.

The Psychodynamic Model

The psychodynamic model coexists with the medical model and does not necessarily contradict it. Since drugs or shock therapy have emerged as effective ways of managing schizophrenia or depression, the psychodynamic model has begun to restrict itself to such areas as the neuroses.

Freud evolved his psychodynamic theories while in the process of treating Viennese women suffering from conversion symptoms. Usually these women had visited one neurologist after another, and none had been found who could cure their complaints. Freud received a tip from a fellow physician, Breuer, that simply letting the patient talk about her fears and concerns had been effective in treating one woman Breuer had seen. Breuer was frightened off from trying it in further patients when the woman fell in love with him and made sexual overtures to him. Freud was somewhat braver than Breuer. Although he had similar experiences with a few of his patients, he was not frightened by their infatuation with him and learned to use it as a way of explaining and interpreting to them their symptoms.

As Freud developed the "talk it through" therapy that was to become the international science of psychoanalysis, he began to develop a conceptual system to explain what he found. Basically, Freudian theory operates on three foundations.

The first of these is the theory of the unconscious. This implies that a large proportion of our behavior arises from sources that we are not consciously aware of. For example, our dreams express unconscious wishes or thoughts which would be unacceptable to us on a conscious level. Slips of the tongue are another way that the unconscious may express itself.

A second foundation of Freudian theory is psychic determinism. This means that nothing in the mind happens by chance or at random. Each thought and action is determined by prior events or thoughts. Practically speaking, this means that adult behavior is strongly influenced by experiences in early childhood.

The third foundation of Freudian theory is the belief in

infantile sexuality. Prudish Victorians, including Freud himself, were quite hesitant to accept this theory, for they preferred to think of young children as innocent and pure. And yet Freud himself, and eventually other psychologists and psychiatrists, began to see overwhelming evidence that young children are indeed aware of their sexuality and can have sexual feelings toward other people such as family members. For example, a young boy can feel a strong attachment to his mother, be quite jealous of his father, and yet fear that his father will punish him by castration for competing with him for maternal love. Freud called such an attachment the "Oedipus complex."

In practice, these theories suggest that psychiatric disorders in adults are due to the continuing pressure of traumatic events or fears which occurred in childhood. Ordinarily, the events producing a neurosis were so traumatic that they were "repressed" and forced to operate unconsciously rather than consciously. Psychoanalytic treatment encourages the patient to "talk it through" so that he finally recovers the unconscious memory which has been repressed and thereby releases the energy which has been tied up through the repression and has produced neurotic behavior. For example, the man who never outgrew his oedipal period will in adult life have trouble establishing healthy normal relationships with male authority figures and with a woman whom he loves. He continues to unconsciously relate to other women as if they were his mother and to men in authority as if they were his father. As he relives the childhood origins of these unconscious feelings, he is eventually able to conquer them.

Psychodynamic theories are not "provable" or "testable" to the same extent that genetic or biochemical hypotheses are. They tend to be more philosophical than quantitative. Nevertheless, psychodynamic theories have been used effectively to understand the workings of the human mind and to treat psychiatric disorders such as hysteria or anxiety neurosis. Until something better has been discovered, they perhaps provide the best explanation for the origin of the neuroses and the best insights concerning methods of treating them.

The Behavioral Model

Behaviorism developed in reaction to the Freudian psychodynamic approach. Behaviorists such as Skinner, Wolpe, or Eysenck argue that the model used by Freud and his patients to understand the human mind was "unscientific." They maintain that the proper study of mankind is human behavior rather than human thought processes. Only that which could be objectively observed and measured is allowed as evidence in understanding or treating psychiatric disorders.

Behaviorism also stands in rebellion against the medical model, with its emphasis on carefully defined diagnostic entities and on determining the cause of illness. Behaviorists believe that pathological behavior is governed by the same rules as those which govern normal behavior. From the point of view of the behaviorist, neurosis and psychosis are simply abnormal behaviors that have been learned in the same way that normal behavior is learned. If they were more flexible or less extreme, they would be indistinguishable from normal behavior.

Behavioral theories also differ from those previously discussed in that they place no great emphasis on the causes of different kinds of behavior. Behavior theory states that a behavior is maintained by an individual because of a learned system of rewards and punishments; for example, the schizophrenic tends to withdraw and to hallucinate because he has learned that by behaving this way he will either gain positive effects or avoid negative ones. From the point of view of the behaviorists, then, treatment simply consists of teaching the individual new behavior. By rewarding the schizophrenic for more normal behavior, such as participating in social activities, and by punishing him for withdrawal, such as by giving him less appetizing meals, they feel they can teach the schizophrenic to function more effectively in society.

Just as the medical model applies most neatly to serious psychiatric disorders such as schizophrenia or depression, and the psychodynamic model applies most neatly to neuroses, the behavioral model is also applicable to certain areas. The behaviorist's emphasis on reinforcing good behavior with rewards and diminishing unacceptable behavior through punishment is useful in child rearing, the management of alcoholism, the treatment of anxiety and phobias, and handling antisocial or criminal behavior. Although it is doubtful that behavioral techniques can cure schizophrenia, many chronically hospitalized schizophrenics have improved in social skills as a result of behavioral modification techniques. Overall, however, it offers more promise as a mode of treatment for specific sorts of disorders than as a general explanation for the cause of psychiatric disorders.

4

Types of Treatment

*No man is an Iland, intire of it selfe;
every man is a peece of the Continent,
a part of the maine: if a Clod bee
washed away by the Sea, Europe is
the lesse, as well as if a Promontorie
were, as well as if a Mannor of thy
friends, or of thine owne were; Any
Mans death diminishes me, because I
am involved in Mankinde. . . .*

DEVOTIONS, JOHN DONNE

Fortunately, as Donne has stated so eloquently, no man *is* an island. Facilities and personnel available to help people with emotional or psychiatric problems have increased enormously in both quality and quantity over the past 30 years. The various types of personnel, facilities, and therapy available are described in this chapter.

What Kind of Help?

The first question often asked by a person who recognizes symptoms of illness in himself or a loved one is: Who should I turn to for help? A variety of types of help are available, and the type needed depends to some extent on the problem involved. In general, the more serious psychiatric disorders such as schizophrenia or depression should almost always be handled by someone with a medical background. Supplementary help may often come from others such as social workers and ministers. The full range of people available to help include the psychiatrist, social worker, clinical psychologist, family doctor, or family minister. Each of these has a different background and different capabilities for helping the person with emotional problems.

A psychiatrist is always a medical doctor or physician who has completed premedical training plus four years of medical school. Thereafter he spends four to five additional years obtaining specialty training in his chosen field of psychiatry by working as a psychiatric resident in an approved training program. This quantity of training is the bare minimum for a person who identifies himself as a psychiatrist. Because the training program in a psychiatric residency also includes some work in neurology, in many areas psychiatrists handle both types of problems, particularly in small towns where no neurologists are available. Likewise, a neurologist may handle psychiatric problems in a small town, for he has received some psychiatric training during his neurology residency. Some psychiatrists choose to take additional specialty training. For example, an additional one to two years are required for specialization in child psychiatry. A person who chooses to emphasize psychoanalysis must spend an additional two to three years working in this area.

The training of the psychiatrist therefore has placed heavy emphasis on medical illness, and the psychiatrist is most likely to follow the medical model. Among the helping figures available, only the psychiatrist (or another person trained medically such as the family doctor or neurologist) is able to hospitalize patients and prescribe medications for them. The psychiatrist is, therefore, particularly suited for dealing with the types of illness which usually require somatic therapy such as depression or schizophrenia. He is also the person to turn to if there is a question concerning an interaction between physical illness and emotional problems—in the case of the elderly individual with an organic brain syndrome, emotional problems complicating cardiac disease, and other such problems which require an understanding of both psychiatry and medicine. Most psychiatrists provide a wider range of services than simply prescribing drugs, however, and most have been trained in working with the various therapies described later in this chapter—behavior therapy, psychotherapy, and group therapy.

Clinical psychologists are also licensed to provide clinical services, either in private practice or in hospitals in conjunction with a physician. The training for a clinical psychologist consists of undergraduate college education plus a masters and usually a Ph.D. degree. The background of the clinical psychologist tends to be more humanistic than medical, although the Ph.D. clinical psychologist does receive training in neuroanatomy, neurophysiology, and neurochemistry. Unless supervised by a physician, a clinical psychologist is unable to prescribe drugs or hospitalize patients. Some clinical psychologists work in conjunction with psychiatrists, providing such services as psychotherapy or psychological testing. Others prefer to work alone in private practice, and generally their services include the range of nonsomatic therapies such as psychotherapy, behavior therapy, and group therapy.

The social worker has usually completed an undergraduate college degree plus a masters program in social work and sometimes a Ph.D. degree. Like the clinical psychologists, their training has not emphasized medical areas, although many social workers who work in conjunction with physicians or hospitals pick up considerable expertise and knowledge in this area, just as the clinical psychologist may. The social worker, because his training emphasizes social and family problems, is particularly well equipped to handle difficulties in these areas. Like the clinical psychologist, the social worker may work alone in private practice or in conjunction with a physician. He may do individual psychotherapy, and many social workers are often very skilled in handling marital problems or doing family therapy.

A family physician is often a good person to turn to initially for evaluation and referral to one of the types of clinicians described above. A person in family practice has completed a bare minimum of premedical education, medical school, and a year of internship. Some are now also completing family practice residencies of three years duration. The ideal family doctor knows the entire family whom he serves and is particularly in tune with their overall needs and problems. A family physician or general practitioner may serve either as a referral source or may himself choose to treat a variety of emotional problems. Few are interested in getting deeply involved in psychotherapy or hospitalizing patients for psychiatric problems. On the other hand, many of the complaints for which patients consult a family physician are emotional in nature, and family doctors are particularly adept at handling mild problems of anxiety and depression either by counseling briefly or by prescribing medication. Family physicians sometimes assume total responsibility for handling hyperactive children or schizophrenics on maintenance medication.

In our present social framework, the clergyman is another person in addition to the family doctor who is well equipped to understand the total family and its problems. Usually, like the family doctor, he has come to know all the family members over a substantial period of time. Therefore, he can be particularly helpful in providing advice about whether sudden changes in behavior are significant and about interpersonal interactions either within the family or the community. Clergymen are primarily trained in theology, but more and more are recognizing their need for specialized training in the counseling role in which they are often placed. Regardless of whether a minister can provide either psychotherapy or medication, he is often well-equipped to provide advice about personal problems or matters of conscience. Further, like the family physician, he may serve as a valuable referral source to a psychiatrist, social worker, clinical psychologist, or family doctor if he recognizes emotional problems of sufficient seriousness that he feels unable to handle them. Often he or the family physician will have more moral authority than anyone else in persuading a family member to seek psychiatric help.

The Various Therapies

DRUG THERAPY. Sedating medications such as phenobarbital, which relax and promote sleep, have been available for many years. These have never been particularly effective in people with significant emotional problems, and they are almost never used today. In 1953 a significant breakthrough in drug therapy for psychiatric illness occurred when chlorpromazine (Thorazine) was placed on the market. This drug, and its later-discovered cousins in the general category known as phenothiazines, is an extremely potent anti-psychotic medication. This group of drugs is used for a variety of problems, including schizophrenia, mania, and organic brain syndromes. Particularly when first introduced, it seemed to produce miracles, for it often diminished delusions and hallucinations, as well as assaultive and combative behavior. Chemical restraints could replace physical restraint, and psychiatric wards became much more pleasant and humane. Further, many patients who had been chronically hospitalized for a number of years improved sufficiently on phenothiazines so that they could be discharged into the community.

Through advances in pharmacology in the past twenty years, a wide variety of phenothiazines and other related drugs are now available. Some of these are more sedating and particularly suitable for patients when they are hostile or combative. Others seem to be more energizing and are used in apathetic withdrawn patients. Psychiatrists can now tailor their chemotherapy to the particular problems of particular patients.

We realize that these drugs cannot cure all psychotic illnesses. Some patients never get completely well on the antipsychotic drugs, but some schizophrenics do recover fully when treated with phenothiazines during an acute episode. Others are able to lead useful and significant lives while continually maintained on low doses of phenothiazines. Usually aggressive behavior, delusions, and hallucinations are the symptoms most amenable to treatment with phenothiazines. The emotional flattening in schizophrenia is perhaps the most difficult symptom to eliminate with drug therapy.

All medications have side effects, and these are often a problem in patients treated with phenothiazines. Perhaps the most common is known as the "Parkinsonian syndrome," a symptom cluster consisting of lack of expression in the face, a shuffling gait, a mild tremor of the hands, and a generalized appearance of rigidity. Some patients experience the side effect known as akathisia, an internal feeling of restlessness and the need to keep their legs moving continually. Sometimes the drugs also cause blurring of vision. If these side effects are troublesome, however, most respond to supplementary anti-Parkinsonian medication.

The antidepressants were discovered in the late 1950s, and to some extent they still seem to be wonder drugs. Like the phenothiazines, a wide battery of antidepressants has been evolved since they were first discovered. Some are more sedating and are particularly useful for patients suffering from anxious or agitated depression. Others are more energizing and tend to be used for apathetic or "retarded" depression. Thus the physician can also tailor antidepressant medication to suit his particular patients. Ordinarily a person suffering from depression does not respond immediately after antidepressants are instituted, however. Depending on the particular medication and the severity of the depression, the drugs may take from one to three weeks to take effect. Thus a person suffering from depression needs careful supervision during this time. Many patients with depression can be managed as outpatients on antidepressant medication, but those who present a serious suicide risk may need to be hospitalized during the interval required for the antidepressants to act. The mechanism for the slowness of this action is not known, but is probably related to being able to build up adequate blood levels of the antidepressant.

Antidepressants, too, have their side effects. Patients often find these particularly unpleasant during the interval while they are waiting for the therapeutic effect of these drugs, and during this period they may need particular support to continue taking the medication. Common side effects include dryness of mouth, hand tremor, constipation, dizziness upon standing up suddenly, and sometimes slowing of the urinary stream. Side effects should always be mentioned to the supervising physician when they are noted, so that he can evaluate whether supplementary therapy is necessary or whether the medication should be changed or readjusted.

Tranquilizers are a third category of drugs currently used, and they are perhaps the most widely used. These medications are most commonly prescribed for symptoms such as anxiety or mild depression. They have been markedly helpful in patients suffering from neurotic problems, since they tend to decrease the inner feelings of pain and discomfort. They are relatively safe drugs with few side effects or hazards. Perhaps the most serious is drowsiness, particularly if they are combined with alcohol. In general, it is best to avoid alcohol or keep its consumption to a bare minimum when one is taking tranquilizers or any of the drugs mentioned above. A second hazard with tranquilizers is physical or emotional dependency. Many patients find these medications so helpful in easing their anxiety that they are hesitant to give them up after the crisis for which they were prescribed

has passed. And indeed some patients do need chronic maintenance on tranquilizers, although this should be avoided
whenever possible. We are beginning to realize that when
taken in sufficiently large quantities over sufficiently long periods of time, patients may develop a physical dependency on
tranquilizers and suffer withdrawal symptoms if they are
abruptly discontinued, just as is the case with alcohol. Therefore, a patient who is taking tranquilizers should always
notify someone of this if he is placed in a position where they
might be abruptly withdrawn.

Several general warnings about drugs should be added.
Physicians always need to know a complete list of the types
and quantities of drugs that their patients are taking. Drug
interactions may be quite complex. For example, a person
suffering from high blood pressure who is placed on antidepressants may receive little benefit from his antihypertensive
medication because its effect is partially negated by the antidepressants. In other cases, effects may be additive, and the
patient taking tranquilizers and drugs for high blood pressure
may find himself heavily sedated. Anyone on medication
should insist that his physician identify the name and
amount to him and should take responsibility himself for
keeping a list of the medications and dosages he is taking.
These should always be presented when a new doctor is
consulted. A second warning concerns the risk of overdose
with any of these medications. Antidepressants, phenothiazines, and tranquilizers are all potent drugs. Phenothiazines
and especially antidepressants can be quite hazardous in people suffering from cardiac problems, and even small overdoses can be fatal. Further, overdose is even more hazardous
in children than adults. One or two pills have been known
to be fatal. These drugs should, therefore, be handled very
carefully in families with small children, kept high up out of
reach, and children should be firmly instructed not to touch
them.

ELECTROTHERAPY. The antidepressants and phenothiazines have diminished the need for electrotherapy—variously known as electrotherapy (ET), electroshock therapy (EST), or electroconvulsive therapy (ECT). Nevertheless, some severe depressions and a few patients with schizophrenia (usually acute schizophrenia) do not respond to medication, and it may be necessary for the physician to prescribe electrotherapy. Further, in some cases electrotherapy may be quicker and more efficient than antidepressants. Unfortunately, media such as films have dramatized electrotherapy in a way to make it appear quite terrifying. It is, in fact, a safe and painless procedure which in some cases may be the only effective therapy available.

The technique for electrotherapy is quite simple. Ordinarily, it is given to hospitalized patients, although it may occasionally be used on an outpatient basis. About a half hour prior to the treatment, the patient is given an injection to relax him and dry up secretions in his nasopharynx. Immediately prior to the treatment he is given a series of medications which first put him to sleep for several minutes and then completely relax all his muscles. The actual treatment consists of passing a small current of electricity between electrodes applied to the temples which stimulates a convulsion similar to that which occurs in patients with epilepsy. Because of the medications given previously, the convulsion is "attenuated" and occurs only in the brain without accompanying body movement. Attenuation of convulsions has markedly decreased the hazards of electrotherapy, which were similar to those of an epileptic seizure—primarily injury to muscles and bones due to the violent movements which occur when an epileptic seizure is not attenuated. The patient wakes up about a minute after the electrotherapy has been applied. Sometimes he suffers from a mild headache, and this ordinarily clears in a few hours.

The primary complaint of patients who receive electrotherapy is the memory loss which occurs. Ordinarily a series of eight treatments is given at intervals of about every other day. The memory loss is cumulative—minimal after the first treatment but relatively troublesome after the last. Memory loss is not permanent, however, and memory usually returns completely within a month to six weeks. No permanent memory loss or intellectual impairment has been found to occur. The number eight is, of course, an average. A physician may chose to give fewer or more depending on the individual patient. Since a course of electrotherapy often can be completed in less than three weeks and a good response is relatively certain, it may be more rapidly effective than drugs, even allowing time for memory loss to clear. Some physicians may, therefore, choose to use it particularly in those people eager to get back to work rapidly.

PSYCHOSURGERY. Psychosurgery is the third of the various types of so-called somatic or physical therapies. Twenty years ago it was widely heralded and publicized as a promising treatment for relieving symptoms in severely disturbed patients. In general, that promise has not been fulfilled and it is now rarely used. Very occasionally, however, it may be helpful. The original procedure, prefrontal lobotomy, was not a particularly delicate or sophisticated surgical technique. Large tracts of white matter in the frontal lobes of the brain were severed, with the result that the individual became much calmer and more manageable but was also even less socially appropriate. Newer techniques involve surgery on very small quantities of white matter, and at present this technique is most commonly used in severe obsessive-compulsive personalities. Very good results have occurred in some cases, but neurosurgeons and psychiatrists both remain extremely cautious about the use of this procedure. Other forms of psychosurgery have also been developed. This includes operations on the thalamus, or pain center of the brain, to relieve severe intractable pain, and on the temporal lobe, to control severe rage attacks or unmanageable seizure disorders.

PSYCHOTHERAPY. Psychotherapy is a general term which refers to a wide range of quite different techniques. They all share the common goal of achieving changes in behavior and attitude through talking, achieving insight, becoming introspective, understanding interactions with other people, or remembering and reliving traumatic moments from the distant past. Drugs may or may not be used in conjunction with psychotherapy, depending on the therapist's point of view. Some psychiatrists or psychologists adhere to a particular school of psychotherapy such as psychoanalysis. Others use all the various forms of psychotherapy and attempt to tailor the type chosen to the individual patient.

The oldest form of psychotherapy is classical psychoanalysis. This is the "talk therapy" discovered by Freud which became an international movement in the early twentieth century and has been a popular and fashionable mode of psychiatric treatment for many years. It is still widely used, particularly on the East Coast, although its popularity is waning.

Classical psychoanalysis by definition involves hourly appointments for a minimum of three days per week. A few analysts will see patients only two days per week and some will require that the analysis occurs five days per week. The treatment lasts for two or three years. The patient ordinarily lies on a couch with the analyst seated behind him and "free associates," which means saying whatever comes into his mind. Freud discovered that this technique was useful in helping patients recover memories and relive experiences which they had repressed because they were too painful. The analyst typically says very little but occasionally makes what is known as an "interpretation." This usually consists of pointing out a repetitive pattern in the patient's life or noting an association between a childhood event and the patient's behavior at present. The goal in psychoanalysis is a greater understanding of one's self and freedom from neurotic emotions and behavior. Most analysts feel that this freedom cannot be achieved through insight alone but that the patient must experience emotional catharsis as he deals with traumatic events.

People who provide psychoanalytic treatment are themselves required to undergo a period of psychoanalysis, and training in psychoanalysis requires about five years beyond the ordinary medical training. Most psychoanalysts are physicians, but a few, known as "lay analysts," have had training in psychology or even the humanities and then undergone psychoanalytic training at a psychoanalytic institute in order to become certified by the American Psychoanalytic Association.

Classical psychoanalysis is appropriate only for a small number of people. In the first place, few can afford the time or money required for the treatment. Secondly, a person who undergoes such intensive self-exploration must be relatively healthy emotionally to begin with, for psychoanalysis itself is painful and traumatic. Because of these limitations in classical psychoanalysis, a variation on it known as psychoanalytic psychotherapy has developed. Ordinarily such therapy is conducted face-to-face rather than with the patient lying on a couch, and more direction or interpretation is given by the therapist. In classical psychoanalysis, the patient is expected to develop a "transference neurosis," which means that he transfers to the therapist emotions which he originally felt for a significant figure in his life such as a parent. If he did not see the therapist face-to-face, the therapist would, therefore, remain a shadowy figure and the "transference would be enhanced." Psychoanalytic psychotherapy places less emphasis on using the development of transference neurosis as a means of treatment, but it does use the valuable and often correct insights of Freud about why people behave and feel as they do. Psychoanalytic psychotherapy also emphasizes remembering and reliving the emotions associated with traumatic past events. Ordinarily psychoanalytic psychotherapy is done for one to two hours a week over the course of a year or two.

In addition, an entire series of briefer psychotherapies has evolved. Most psychiatrists are willing to see patients for only one or two hours in order to provide assistance and advice concerning a crisis in their lives that they may be facing. This brief psychotherapy tends to be quite direct and to the point, with strong emphasis on looking at the present and the future rather than the past. On the other hand, short-term psychotherapy may consist of a series of hourly appointments on a weekly basis over the course of two or three months. Again the therapist will be quite directive, will look at the present primarily, but will use past behavior as a way of understanding how the patient has gotten himself in difficulty and how he may get himself back out of it. In general, the briefer psychotherapies aim primarily at achieving insight and thereby effecting change in behavior. Another variation of briefer psychotherapy is known as "supportive psychotherapy." This is used most frequently for patients suffering from intermittent depressive illnesses or mild neurosis. Such patients are seen for an hour every few weeks, every month, or every few months, and the main goal is to analyze the present and future and to provide practical supportive advice. Supportive psychotherapy is often combined with drug therapy.

Group therapy is one of the more recent developments in psychotherapy. It is popular in the Midwest as well as on the West Coast, where a group of widely publicized institutes has developed and evolved a variety of techniques. The essential ingredient for group therapy is assembling a number of people together, usually from five to ten, under the leadership of a trained individual. Group members are then encouraged to interact with one another and share their insights and awareness about one another's behavior. Depending on the goal of the group, the leader may assume either an active or a passive role. In a situation known as a "T Group," the leader normally remains relatively inactive. T Groups are in theory composed of normal individuals who wish to meet with others like themselves in order to expand their awareness of their emotions and behavior. The goal is enrichment rather than change. On the other hand, therapy groups are composed of people considered to have some type of psychiatric disorder, ordinarily problems such as neuroses or drug and alcohol dependence, and the aim is to effect changes in their behavior through evaluation, criticism, and analysis by other members of the group. The group leader may become actively involved if he feels this will enhance the therapeutic role. In therapy groups, great emphasis is placed on developing group loyalty and cohesiveness and on using group pressure as a means of effecting change.

Another form of therapy currently available is known as family therapy. This type of therapy is particularly useful for problems which involve the entire family, such as pathological interactions between parents and/or children which may lead to drinking problems, adolescent rebellion, or marital conflict. The entire family is seen as a group for family therapy, and children and parents are encouraged to comment candidly on one another's behavior in order to identify the nature of their pathological interactions. Once these are identified, the therapist assists the family members in finding new ways to relate to one another. Family therapy is usually conducted by psychiatrists or social workers working either alone or as a team.

BEHAVIOR THERAPY. Behavior therapy grows out of the theoretical constructs concerning the origins of psychiatric illness already described in the third chapter. Like other therapies, at its outset behavior therapy was widely heralded as a rapid and effective means of treating psychiatric problems which had been refractory to other forms of treatment. With time we have come to realize that it may perhaps be no quicker and that it is not as widely effective as was hoped, but nevertheless, it remains a valuable mode of treatment for some disorders.

Negative conditioning is perhaps the most commonly used technique of behavior therapy. It is used most frequently for alcoholism and homosexuality, two problems with which psychiatry has had little success in the past. If negative conditioning is used as a treatment technique for homosexuality, the individual seeking treatment must make a definite choice that he wishes to change his sexual orientation. Most psychiatrists consider homosexuality a problem only if a particular individual himself identifies it as a problem and wishes to change. Techniques of negative conditioning ordinarily involve putting the patient in the situation which he wishes to learn to dislike. For example, the alcoholic is given liquor to drink or the male homosexual is shown photographs of other men whom he finds particularly attractive. While in this situation, the patient is then given an unpleasant stimulus. For the treatment of alcoholism, this is often a drug which will make him vomit after the ingestion of alcohol. For the homosexual the stimulus is usually a mild but unpleasant electric shock applied to his hand. Depending on the problem and its severity, a series of treatments is used until the patient himself feels that he has learned to dislike alcohol or find other members of his sex physically unappealing.

Another form of behavior therapy is known as reciprocal inhibition. This is often used for phobias or anxiety. The patient is first taught relaxation therapy—how to systematically and consistently relax various muscle groups in his body until he feels a pleasant state of total relaxation. Once he has learned techniques for relaxation, he is then placed near the situation or stimulus which evokes his fear or anxiety. While in the situation he is then requested to assume the relaxed state of mind and body that he has learned to produce himself. Gradually he learns to gain control over the fear or anxiety through consciously relaxing himself in its presence.

Treatment Facilities

Treatment facilities are basically of two types—outpatient and inpatient. Outpatient treatment facilities include individual physicians' offices, clinics, and a variety of community facilities. Inpatient treatment invariably occurs in hospitals, of which various types are available.

Evaluation on an outpatient basis is the logical place to begin for most people seeking psychiatric help. Some people are lucky enough to have a knowledgeable family physician, minister, or lawyer who can immediately sense the types of problems and recommend the appropriate source from whom to seek help. Most people, however, are not this lucky, and the decision as to where to go can be quite difficult. Facilities vary from one community to another, depending on community size and level of medical sophistication. Thanks to a strong mental health movement established in many areas through the national leadership of a man named Clifford Beers, himself a manic-depressive who wrote an eloquent account describing his experiences with the illness *(A Mind That Found Itself)*, some communities have excellent mental health centers. In others only private facilities will be available.

The typical community mental health center is staffed by a psychiatrist, a psychologist, and a social worker at the bare minimum. Larger community mental health centers will have several workers in each category on a full-time basis, while in smaller ones the psychiatrist may work in the community facility part-time while involved in teaching or private practice activities during the remainder of his time. Community mental health centers are funded by individual states or counties and tend to be community and service-oriented. Ordinarily, treatment at a mental health center is much less expensive than with a private psychiatrist. Community mental health centers can usually be identified simply through telephone book listings, and if you are unable to determine whether or not one is available in your area, you can probably obtain this information through a local social service agency. Because they are service-oriented and try to reach a large number of people, community mental health centers ordinarily do not provide extensive psychotherapy. They are most useful for evaluation, crisis intervention, and brief or supportive psychotherapy, as well as the management of medication. Community mental health centers usually do not have inpatient facilities of their own, and patients requiring hospitalization are referred from them either to private hospitals or to state hospitals.

Some communities also have family service agencies instead of or in addition to community mental health centers. Family service agencies are typically staffed by psychologists and social workers. Like the mental health centers, they can usually be found by looking under the appropriate heading in a phone book. Some of these are church-oriented, and your minister may know about whether one is available in your area or not. Family service agencies tend to specialize in marital and divorce counseling, family therapy, and youth and drug problems. Like the mental health center, they are service-oriented and provide short-term counseling rather than extensive psychotherapy. They usually do not have a psychiatrist working within the agency, although one may be available to them on a consultant basis. Management of patients on psychoactive drugs is usually outside their scope.

Private treatment facilities tend to be available much more extensively. In a moderate-size midwestern town, an outpatient diagnostic evaluation ordinarily costs approximately fifty dollars and psychotherapy sessions cost approximately thirty-five dollars an hour. These tend to be higher in larger cities and on either coast. More and more insurance companies, however, are extending their coverage to include outpatient treatment of all types, including psychiatric treatment. The primary advantage of private psychiatric treatment is continuity of care and personal involvement by the physician. Like all physicians, psychiatrists vary in skill and personality. Further, within a particular community psychiatrists also tend to vary in point of view. Some psychiatrists are much more medically oriented and tend to concentrate their practice on drug management and electrotherapy with a minimal emphasis on psychotherapy. Others tend to specialize particularly in psychotherapy and may not wish to take on patients requiring extensive hospitalization. Tactful enquiry of a potentially knowledgeable source, such as a family friend or minister, may be helpful in indicating which private psychiatrist might be most appropriate for a particular problem. If you are unable to obtain the information, it is not inappropriate to phone a psychiatrist's office and obtain from his secretary information concerning fees, types of treatment provided, and whether the psychiatrist has hospital facilities available to him.

Whatever type of outpatient treatment you seek, any good facility will make every effort possible to respect your privacy and to keep your records confidential. All psychiatrists are ethically required to treat anything they are told as privileged communication except under the special circumstance that their records are subpoenaed on court order. In practice, this means that a psychiatrist will not reveal what a patient has told him without obtaining specific permission from the patient himself. If you ask a psychiatrist about a friend's or relative's condition, he may be rather vague and evasive because of this rule of confidentiality. If the patient has agreed that he can talk freely with a relative or friend, then ordinarily the psychiatrist will do so. In come cases, such as marital discord or adolescent problems, confidentiality is usually an absolute necessity if the psychiatrist is to make any headway at all with the patient. Many private offices are carefully set up to protect the patient's privacy. A series of waiting rooms may be available so that patients do not see one another come and go. If you have a particular concern about privacy, you should communicate this to the psychiatrist you are seeing and usually he will try his best to respect your wishes.

INPATIENT FACILITIES. People who are unfamiliar with psychiatric wards usually accept a stereotyped view. A person may imagine psychiatric wards as snake pits—dark, crowded, dismal places where unkempt people pound the walls or sit in a stupor all day long. At the other extreme, some people envision psychiatric hospitals as full of golden sunlight and cheerful sweet-faced nurses who move through bright modern surroundings tending the needs of patients who are inspired to get well simply by the beauty of the atmosphere. In fact, psychiatric hospitals or wards are rarely like either of those extremes, but rather tend to fall somewhere between them.

Basically there are three types of hospitals which specialize in the care of psychiatric patients. These are private hospitals, university hospitals, and state hospitals. State hospitals have improved remarkably over the years, and few, if any, meet the "snake pit" stereotype. Some are housed in quite old facilities, however, and making them beautiful and modern would be quite difficult. Further, state hospitals tend to house at least some patients requiring chronic hospitalization who have not responded to any form of treatment and may remain in the hospital the remainder of their lives. Such patients are almost never found in university or private hospitals. Current thinking in most state hospitals now is that even these patients benefit, however, from mingling with patients who have a better prognosis. They are no longer hidden on "back wards," and therefore they are definitely visible to anyone who visits a friend or relative in a state hospital. State hospitals, as the name implies, are financed by state government, and therefore treatment there is usually less expensive.

University hospitals are teaching hospitals. Facilities vary from old fashioned to very modern depending on the wealth and age of the particular university. Such hospitals are ordinarily staffed by permanent faculty members who may work in the hospital on either a full or part-time basis and by a group of resident physicians in training who care for patients under the supervision of the faculty. Most university hospitals handle both state and private patients. In some cases university facilities exist as completely separate hospitals, and in others they represent a wing or a substantial area of a general hospital. Private hospitals devoted exclusively to psychiatric care are not numerous, but a few very fine ones exist. They tend to be relatively expensive, but insurance coverage increases the availability of such facilities to larger numbers of people. In most cases, however, a psychiatrist seen on a private basis will have hospital privileges on a psychiatric ward within a general hospital.

Routines on psychiatric wards vary from hospital to hospital. In general, physicians, nurses, and aides make a strong effort to keep patients active and busy. Patients usually wear street clothes in most psychiatric facilities, and in many, nurses and attendants also wear street clothing rather than white uniforms. Psychiatric nurses often assume a significant role in counseling patients and providing supportive therapy during their hospital stay. Most hospitals provide some form of recreational activity on a daily basis, such as attending movies, having parties or song fests, or working together on an artistic project. In many hospitals patients often have private rooms, and they gather for meals or recreational activities in a common living room or dining area. Some hospitals continue to have "locked wards," while others do not. In general, these wards occur in those hospitals which care for severely disturbed patients, since they could become a danger to themselves and others if permitted to leave freely without supervision. Even on such "locked wards," however, the majority of patients are permitted to come and go at will simply by asking someone to unlock the door. Facilities which handle acutely disturbed patients often have an area where patients are kept alone in order to quiet them down when they are behaving violently.

Although most people imagine psychiatric hospitals as gloomy or violent, these hospitals in fact tend to be relatively cheerful and pleasant places, even when the buildings themselves are not ultramodern. Both patients and their relatives are often pleasantly surprised when they find out what psychiatric facilities are really like. Patients, in fact, usually show a great sense of relief on being hospitalized, since they know they will be protected from their frightening or harmful impulses. Some patients even grow so fond of the hospital that they must be protected against the condition known as "hospital dependency," which refers to the feeling that they could not maintain a satisfactory life outside the hospital. Psychiatric patients are sometimes popularly imagined as pitiful people locked away in institutions for life, but in fact the thrust of modern psychiatry is to prevent hospitalizations whenever possible, to make it as brief as possible when it does occur, and to prevent as many patients as possible from remaining chronically hospitalized.

5

How Friends and Relatives Can Help

So faith, hope, love abide, these three; but the greatest of these is love.

1 CORINTHIANS 13:13

Good psychiatric help and effective drugs and other forms of treatment are crucial to recovery or remission of symptoms in psychiatric disorders. But the help that friends and relatives can provide is perhaps even more crucial. Philosophers of the past have commented that man is "a thinking animal" or "a political animal." One might also add that man is a spiritual animal. As all these statements indicate, human beings are characterized by their need for one another and their need for a feeling of purpose or meaning in their lives. They need faith, hope, and love, but most of all love. Psychiatrists and medications can help patients alleviate their symptoms. But friends and relatives can help them find faith, hope, and love.

Recognizing Symptoms

The first reaction of a friend or relative to the development of symptoms in a loved one is often a refusal to recognize symptoms. To psychiatrists, this is the familiar "mental mechanism" of "denial." Denial is both a great source of

79

comfort and a great deceiver. Essentially, it is a refusal to recognize warning signals because they are too frightening or too painful. It is denial, for example, which prevents the heavy smoker with a chronic cough and difficulty breathing from giving up smoking before he develops emphysema or cancer. Or it is denial which prevents women from going in for annual pap smears or recognizing the danger signals of carcinoma of the cervix such as unusual bleeding. None of us wishes to recognize something as painful as the potentiality or reality of illness and death. When denial prevents people from recognizing symptoms, it is a great danger and a great deceiver. Nevertheless, it can also be a great source of comfort at times, particularly in the case of a person who has a terminal illness but wishes to go on living as happy and normal a life as possible prior to his death.

Just as people avoid recognizing the symptoms of physical illness in themselves or others as long as possible, so too they often avoid recognizing symptoms of psychiatric illness. Bill, for example, who was slowly developing symptoms of schizophrenia began to believe he was possessed by witches and began to hear their voices talking to him and to see them appearing before him. Terribly frightened by this experience, he told his parents about it, and they replied that it was his imagination or a bad dream. He again told them about it two or three times more, but when he received the same reply, he finally decided to keep the experience to himself. It was finally called to everyone's attention when he broke into a church and defaced the altar when the commands from the witches became irresistible. Perhaps if Bill had received treatment when the first warning symptoms were communicated to his parents, he and society might have been spared at least some of the consequences of his illness. It is, of course, only natural to hope that, if one closes his eyes and ignores the symptoms, they will go away. Occasionally this happens, but not often.

You may be asking yourselves: how do I know there

really is a problem? Some warning signals are so flagrant that they should never be denied. Bill's hallucinations of witches, described to his parents with great fear and emotion, represent an example of a very obvious warning signal. So, too, is the expression of a desire to commit suicide in a person who has also been clearly despondent. In general, it is easier to determine that a person definitely needs help if the problem is either quite serious or quite acute. More specifically, it is easier to make decisions in illnesses such as depression, schizophrenia, or mania.

Sometimes a person coming down with a psychiatric illness directly expresses his symptoms and asks for help. If this occurs, the problem is relatively simple. More often, a friend or relative must himself assume responsibility for recognizing the meaning of changes in behavior. He may simply notice that Mike has become secretive and uncommunicative. When people talk to him his answers are brief and evasive. He may withdraw to his bedroom and be very seclusive, or he may simply sit apathetically in a chair and stare into space. Molly may show little interest in food and begin to lose weight. She may toss and turn in bed at night or complain that she can no longer sleep. She may begin to run herself down, alluding to her worthlessness or sinfulness. Such people may be in very great pain and wish treatment, but they may be afraid to ask for it because they fear criticism, rejection, or mockery. It is indeed a sad situation if the denial system of a sick person and that of a loved one interact with one another so that both avoid getting help for the suffering person. If you notice symptoms like these, *ask* in a kindly way about the person's behavior. Indicate that you feel they may need help and that you will give them support in seeking it.

You should be aware that if a person is very ill, he may not realize his need for help. For example, a person who is very depressed may feel so worthless and guilt-ridden that he actually wishes to die and considers it his due. He may feel that total abandonment and neglect is all that he deserves. Therefore, if asked whether he wishes help, he will probably refuse it. In such a case, if you recognize that symptoms of depression are present as they have been previously described, then you have a moral obligation to help him against his wishes. Similar lack of insight about need for treatment occurs in people suffering from schizophrenia or mania, and in the latter illness in particular it may be difficult to persuade the person of his need for treatment.

In the case of illnesses which develop more slowly, such as neurosis or alcoholism, the sudden and dramatic development of symptoms which require treatment is more unlikely. In these cases, therefore, it is more difficult to evaluate when there really is a problem. If in doubt, you should encourage your relative or friend to obtain a psychiatric evaluation and leave the decision about further treatment to him and the psychiatrist involved.

Seeking Treatment

Your role in helping your loved one obtain treatment will vary depending on the nature of the problem. If he is very ill, you may have to take the initiative. If the problem is milder, he will of course be able to make the appointment himself, although your encouragement and support can be of considerable consolation to him. The extent to which you will be involved in the initial appointment will also depend on the nature of the problem and the preferences of the doctor or facility. Some facilities use a team approach. The doctor will see the patient, while a social worker will obtain a supplementary history from an accompanying relative. In other facilities the doctor may wish to see the patient alone.

Once the initial evaluation has been completed, the physician consulted should be permitted to determine what your role in treatment will be. If your relative is significantly depressed, for example, but the physician elects to handle the problem initially on an outpatient basis, he may wish to have you quite actively involved. He may ask you to make sure the patient takes his medication, to watch him closely for the risk of suicide, to help him become more active and interested in things, or to report improvement or worsening of symptoms. On the other hand, he may have some important reason for requesting that you remain minimally involved. If this occurs, you should not take it personally or think that the doctor does not value your opinion. Ordinarily, this simply means that the doctor needs to establish a close relationship with the patient and that communicating with relatives might handicap this relationship. In some cases the doctor may ask that you have a continuing relationship with a social worker or psychologist while he continues to see the patient. In other cases, the doctor may ask to see both you and your relative together or the entire family together for family therapy.

Relatives are placed in a difficult position if they themselves feel that a loved one needs treatment and he in turn refuses. If this situation occurs, you have several options available. You may make the first appointment for yourself and describe your relative's symptoms to the doctor and let him advise you further as to whether or not you should insist that your relative come in. You may enlist the help of a valued friend, minister, or lawyer and have another person join with you in persuading your loved one to seek treatment. If the problems seem severe enough, you have a moral obligation to insist on treatment for him, since the consequences of untreated psychiatric illness can obviously be serious.

Your doctor may recommend hospitalization if the illness is severe. He will usually indicate to you how actively he wishes you to be involved in visiting the patient. Most hospitals have some regulations about visiting hours and who may see the patient. These are usually rather liberal, but if the patient is somewhat disturbed, visiting may be restricted until he improves. Patients are often quite fearful of hospitalizations. This is only a natural reaction. People fear entering a hospital for treatment of a physical illness such as an ulcer, and psychiatric hospitalization also has an element of irrational fear associated with it because of the unenlightened attitude some people have about psychiatric illness. Therefore, you should support and encourage your loved one as much as possible. Usually you will help him by accompanying him to the hospital. Most hospitals have guidelines about what type of clothing and toilet articles he should bring with him, and you will want to help him get the appropriate necessities together.

Sometimes patients refuse hospitalization. This places a painful responsibility upon his relatives. Of course, no physician can force a patient to enter a hospital against his will. He can only recommend that the patient needs hospitalization. If the patient refuses and the risk to his life or the lives of others is significant, then his closest relative is usually asked to sign him into the hospital against his wishes. This is legally known as a commitment. Relatives are often hesitant about committing a patient. They fear he may feel that they have rejected him or mistreated him. Usually after the patient recovers, however, he is grateful to his loved ones for making the decision to help him.

Handling Your Own Feelings

Recognizing the symptoms of psychiatric disorder developing in a loved one is a terrifying experience. For example, your husband or wife's personality may change before your very eyes. A familiar lifetime companion may seem a different person. Depression may cause a vigorous active person to waste away as if consumed by a fatal illness. A teenager stricken with schizophrenia may change from a happy, intelligent, and well-adjusted youngster into a troubled, confused, and tormented person who seems to hold only a poignant shadow of dwindling promise. One may suddenly realize that the evening drink or the cocktail party circuit has turned into a destructive dependency which is crippling a spouse physically and mentally. Or a loved one may suddenly become paranoid, expressing frightening and irrational delusions about how others are trying to attack or poison him. Sometimes the loved one will include members of his family in his delusional system and accuse them of turning against him as well. Disappointment, heartbreak, bitterness, and fear may begin to haunt the relatives of people with psychiatric illness.

You take the first step in handling these feelings when you recognize the symptoms and encourage your loved one to obtain treatment. His doctor may be willing to discuss these reactions with you. Most of the time, however, the "normal" relative is expected by the doctor to carry his responsibilities bravely and without a good deal of advice or support. Many times relatives are able to do this. Family members unite together to console and advise one another, or close friends may offer much-needed encouragement. With the partial disintegration of family life in our era, which means that various family members may be scattered all over the United States and people are frequently on the move, sometimes people do find themselves forced to handle the development of illness in a loved one without comfort or support from friends or relatives. If this should happen, and if you feel the stress becoming intolerable, you should not hesitate to seek someone out to talk with. This may be someone outside the medical field, such as a minister, or you may wish your relative's physician to see you formally or to refer you to another physician or social worker with whom you can talk. In spite of their professional expertise, psychiatrists sometimes forget how difficult it may be for relatives to handle their feelings about illness in a loved one. It does not hurt to remind them.

Whether you talk to someone about them or not, you will notice yourself developing feelings about your relative's illness which you may find troubling. For example, you may become very impatient with a relative who is severely depressed. Quite often, a husband or wife may feel that if only their spouse would get up and do something, the spouse would feel better. They may feel a very understandable but misguided desire to scold or berate their spouse. This will, of course, only worsen the person's feeling of guilt and worthlessness, and so such scolding should be avoided. Or you may become very angry and frustrated with a relative suffering from symptoms of psychiatric illness.

Schizophrenics, in particular, often have an apparent "method in their madness,"—a playful or teasing behavior which seems designed to irritate. For example, they may answer questions obliquely and insultingly, or they may become dirtier and more dilapidated if encouraged repeatedly to wash themselves. Psychiatrists call this trait "negativism," and it, like the apathy of depression, is part of the illness. Neither the apathetic depressive nor the negativistic schizophrenic really wants to be irritating. He simply cannot help it. You, as a loving relative, also cannot help feeling irritated. You will inevitably have feelings toward your relative which you find unpleasant. I can only stress that it is normal to feel this way. No one is saintly enough to deal with really sick people without having such reactions, and you should not feel guilty about them. On the other hand, of course, you should not let such feelings get in the way of an important relationship. Recognizing that such feelings are natural and normal is helpful in learning to handle them and in keeping them from interfering with the relationship.

Being Supportive

Once you have learned to recognize your impatient or angry feelings as normal, you will be better able to support or assist your loved one in his recovery. Most relatives want to be as helpful as possible, but they are never quite sure what they should do. Perhaps the most basic thing the relative of a psychiatric patient can do for his loved one is to reaffirm his love and loyalty. He should indicate from time to time that he is ready to help whenever needed and that the illness will not interfere with their relationship.

Sometimes relatives are not sure about how much advice they should give to the patient. It is a good idea to talk this over with the patient's physician at some point. Ordinarily, a simple guideline is: Don't be afraid to listen to the patient and respond to his thoughts, feelings, or behavior, but also don't try to play psychotherapist yourself. Usually relatives are too close to the patient to make objective interpretations. Sometimes common sense will serve as a guideline. For example, if a patient persists in talking in detail about his sinfulness and guiltiness, when it is perfectly obvious to the observer that he is not a great sinner, this usually means that he wants to be consoled or reassured and thereby in a sense "absolved." It certainly does no harm to positively reassure patients that they are good people, good husbands, good wives, good fathers, or good mothers.

Don't be discouraged if your relative does not respond to a substantial amount of encouragement, however. Patients do need love and loyalty in an abundance, but ordinarily this alone will not "cure" them. If it would, there would be no need for medications or psychotherapy. It is difficult for relatives to continue being encouraging and supportive when they get little positive feedback from the patient about their therapeutic effectiveness. But even if the relative does not respond immediately or even for several months, he usually responds eventually. At some point, as he improves, he will recognize and appreciate your loyalty. In addition to indicating your continued love, you can be supportive to your relative in other ways as well. If he finds the side effects of prescribed medications troubling, you can remind him that these, to some extent, are indications that the medication is working.

If an elderly person with an organic brain syndrome or a younger person who has had electrotherapy has trouble with his memory, you can assist by filling in gaps for him and reorienting him when he is confused. Handling paranoid delusions can be particularly difficult. One does not wish to encourage the delusion, but on the other hand, one does not wish to anger the patient by arguing about them. Ordinarily, a patient cannot be "talked out" of his delusions. It is usually best to avoid replying when the patient discusses them or to indicate frankly that you can see how the patient might feel that way but that you disagree and then drop the matter.

Recognizing Relapses

A final way that the relatives of people who suffer from the vast gamut of psychiatric illnesses can help is by remaining alert for the symptoms of relapse. Although discouraging for patient and loved one alike, relapses are in some respects easier than initial episodes of illness. At least the second or third time around, both patient and relatives have a better understanding of what is happening and have learned some resources for handling the situation. In the case of an initial episode, relatives are usually frightened and use denial. If they recognize the possibility that a relapse may occur, they are usually very careful about evaluating symptoms and seeking treatment immediately if symptoms do recur. In general, the sooner psychiatric illnesses are treated, the better the prognosis. Particularly in the case of illnesses such as depression, but also in the case of schizophrenia, early recognition of symptoms and increasing or reinstituting medication may avert a hospitalization.

Certain psychiatric illnesses are characterized by having a relapsing and remitting course. If relatives know that their loved one has such an illness, they should be particularly alert for the possibility of relapse. Those illnesses which are particularly characterized by relapses and remissions include mania, depression, acute schizophrenia, alcoholism, and drug abuse. To say that these illnesses tend to be relapsing and remitting *does not* mean that relapses are inevitable, however. Each individual has his own characteristic course and pattern. Many people who experience a single episode of each of these illnesses or problems recover completely with treatment and never relapse. Others may have a single relapse, whereas a few have frequent relapses. No one can say what the future holds for a particular patient. Even in the patients who relapse, however, the future is certainly brighter if they have a supportive and enlightened relative standing by to recognize their symptoms and to offer them help in obtaining treatment.

Religion and Psychiatry: The Fourth Dimension

. . . men must learn by suffering
Drop by drop in sleep upon the heart
Falls the laborious memory of pain,
Against one's will comes wisdom.
The grace of the gods is forced on us
Throned inviolably

AGAMEMNON, AESCHYLUS

Traditionally, psychiatry views man in terms of three dimensions—his relationship with himself; his relationship with other people; and his relationship with his surroundings and the physical world. These three dimensions of man have been the subject of previous chapters. Unfortunately, the fourth dimension, his relationship to the supranatural or spiritual, is often ignored or neglected by psychiatrists. This neglect is puzzling and paradoxical, for psychiatry is the most philosophical and humane of all the medical disciplines, and the illnesses it confronts are ones which often blight the human spirit in addition to the mind and emotions. One can only explain the neglect as a byproduct of the pervasive philosophical materialism of the twentieth century and note with hope that existential psychiatry, which does see man as more than a physical being, is receiving more and more attention in psychiatric circles. Man's fourth dimension, his relationship with the supranatural or spiritual, is the subject of this chapter.

The Problem of Moral Responsibility

One of the most difficult issues which both religion and psychiatry must face is the problem of moral responsibility. The Freudian approach in particular has stressed the impact of early childhood on adult behavior. The medical model suggests that many psychiatric illnesses are caused by derangements in body or brain chemistry. In either case, there is an implication that the person suffering from a psychiatric disorder "can't help it." But, on the other hand, such a point of view is prone to lead to an attitude of defeatism or apparently condone morally irresponsible behavior. The following examples illustrate the problem.

> As Mrs. Jones visits her psychiatrist, she gradually realizes that she relates to other people in shallow and immature ways. As she grew up, her feelings and behavior were shaped by cruel rejecting parents who rarely displayed love. Small successes received mocking comments about their lack of importance or the admonition that she really ought to have been able to achieve more. If she failed at something, this was taken as a personal reflection on her family and her parents, and she was sharply criticized. Little gestures of affection such as a good night kiss on being tucked into bed or an invitation to crawl up on her father's knee for a moment were never given. Consequently, she was taught to expect rejection continually and was never able to experience real feelings of trust for other people. Now she is unable

to leave herself open or to give to others. She finds receiving is much easier, and she believes that one had better grab whatever love substitutes one can find, such as food or fine clothing, whenever one can. She lives in a comfortable middle-class home now, is married, and has several children. Continual snacking gives her a weight problem, while fear of physical or emotional closeness gives her a sexual problem. She is jealous of her husband's secretaries and continually accuses him of infidelity. Inability to reach out to other adults gives her an interpersonal problem. She rarely invites people into her home and is unable to show spontaneous signs of friendship. Small wonder that she is lonely, depressed, and sometimes self-pitying.

Mrs. Jones is a tormented, unhappy, fearful and self-centered person. In part, she is living by reaction patterns which she learned as a means of survival during her childhood. Judged from the point of view of most religions, her behavior is not admirable, but it was in part determined by her upbringing. Can she be considered morally responsible?

Mr. Smith is a paranoid schizophrenic. His illness makes him terribly sensitive to rebuffs from other people, and at times when he feels they are "against" him he strikes out with hostility and anger. He is emotionally quite cold and is aloof, superior, and overly stilted and formal to his associates. Although he rarely mentions it, he believes that he is the victim of a conspiracy against his life and well-being which is masterminded by the FBI and CIA, who follow him, harass him, and sometimes secretly enter his home or office and examine his possessions and business records. If someone presses him too hard, or if he becomes too ill, there is always a chance that he may break down completely and commit an act of violence. His thoughts and behavior are in part determined by a complex interaction between his environment and his brain chemistry. Can he be considered morally responsible?

These are difficult questions, both morally and legally. The law is clearer on the matter than ethics, however. The law would consider the neurotic Mrs. Jones completely responsible for her behavior, while the psychotic Mr. Smith would probably be considered "not guilty by reason of insanity." In terms of religious ethics, it is in one sense very cruel to consider either fully responsible, since the behavior of both has been shaped in part by factors which they are unable to control. On the other hand, Mrs. Jones certainly still has free will at any particular moment, and she can make a conscious choice to surmount her neurotic childhood. To a large extent, in fact, she can only benefit from psychotherapy if she is considered fully responsible for her behavior. And therefore the pragmatic and sensible course is to treat her as if she is responsible, although in a compassionate and non-judgmental way.

To some extent this point of view also applies to Mr. Smith. It is therapeutically more effective to consider him responsible for his day to day activities, but aberrant behavior must be regarded much more tenderly in his case. For, to the extent that his illness blinds his insight and reason, he does not truly have free will. And ultimately only God can determine the extent to which either Mrs. Jones or Mr. Smith is to be held accountable. We human beings usually behave more effectively in moral matters if we leave judgment to God and use his mercy and grace as our guidelines when attempting to improve interactions with society.

The Problem of Evil

Even if we leave judgment to God, the presence of psychiatric illness (like the presence of all illness in the world) raises another issue, at least if we follow the medical model and consider the more serious psychiatric disorders as ultimately subtle forms of physical affliction which manifest themselves in the emotional or behavioral spheres. That is the problem of evil: How can a just and loving God permit the torments of illness, particularly those which affect the mind, to afflict mankind when as an omnipotent being he has the power to destroy illness. Or, as the victim of mental illness and his loved ones might phrase the question: Why have we been given this burden to bear? Why must we suffer in this way? What is its meaning for us?

The problem of evil is a subtle theological problem which has been examined by thoughtful men and women for centuries. One could not hope to add much to their theological explanations—that suffering was introduced into the world by man, not God, at the time of the Fall; that suffering tests man's mettle and his love for God; that suffering purifies and leads to wisdom; that suffering leads to compassion for others who suffer; that suffering is the just reward for all men, for all are sinful. Some of these explanations are more convincing or comforting than others, and for the person suffering from psychiatric illness it is perhaps most valuable to focus upon those which stress the positive qualities which grow from suffering.

In the first place, people for many years have suspected that psychosis can for some people be a regenerative or insight-provoking experience. Shakespeare portrays in *King Lear* the way in which Lear grows in maturity and understanding through the course of his madness and emerges again to sanity somehow purified and redeemed. Anton Boisen, a catatonic schizophrenic who has written several books about his experience with psychosis, has said:

> . . . an acute schizophrenic episode assumes the character of a religious experience. It becomes an attempt at thoroughgoing reorganization, beginning at the very center of one's being, an attempt which tends either to

make or break the personality. . . . It was necessary for me to pass through the purgatorial fires of a horrifying psychosis before I could set foot in my promised land of creative activity.

Out of the Depths,
(New York: Harpers, 1960,
pp. 205, 208)

Others have described psychotic illness as potentially a positive disintegration which must precede a creative reintegration in which new insights are both achieved and fully understood. Seen in this way, a psychotic experience may somehow be akin to a mystical experience. Speaking as a psychiatrist who has dealt with many psychotic individuals, I feel that there are less perilous and painful ways to achieve new insights, but nevertheless one cannot ignore those who testify to the value of psychotic experience. And one cannot help but be grateful and hopeful that the potentiality for growth through illness may exist.

Such severe psychotic breaks are fortunately not common. The vast majority of people who experience psychiatric disorders suffer from milder or less crippling forms—the depressions, neuroses, and adjustment problems previously described. These people in particular have a significant potentiality for learning and growing through their experience with suffering. The depressive and the neurotic suffer great emotional pain. Yet, many respond to it by having greater compassion for others who suffer rather than by feeling bitterness or anger. Often working with their illness prompts them to reorganize their lives so that they can use their understanding of suffering to reach out and help others—through volunteer work, through their professional lives, or through their personal lives. Thus many are able to turn their weaknesses into strengths and use their own experience of pain to alleviate the pain of others. In this way, the problem of evil is at least partially resolved. Some good does come out of evil.

The Problem of Guilt:
Can One Be Too Religious?

St. Paul has phrased the fundamental human dilemma with painful clarity in Romans 7:18-19: "I can will what is right, but I cannot do it. For I do not do the good I want, but the evil I do not want is what I do." Human sinfulness and weakness are facts of human nature. Recognition that, as long as he depends upon himself alone, man will remain frail and fallen is the beginning of wisdom from the point of view of Judaeo-Christian tradition, for that recognition will turn the individual toward dependence upon his Creator. Psychiatrists also deal with the fact of human weakness on a daily basis. Some patients are all too painfully aware of their sinfulness, and their preoccupation with their sense of evil paralyzes their capacity to improve. Others seem to need to become more aware of the ways in which their selfish or cruel behavior creates misery for those around them. In attempting to help people suffering from such problems, psychiatrists are only assuming in the secular sphere a role which clergymen have carried for centuries. What is the relationship between psychiatric illness and feelings of guilt? Is a sense of sin always valuable, or can guilt feelings sometimes be excessive?

Through an accident of history, psychiatry has seemed to emphasize that a preoccupation with guilt is dangerous. Psychiatry as a medical science was born during the Victorian era, an age notable for its puritanism, hypocrisy, and emphasis on works and the work ethic. Reacting against this, many psychiatrists began to stress the oppressive and dangerous effects of overharsh and punitive childrearing, puritanical attitudes toward sexuality, and a morbid preoccupation with matters of conscience. At that time, such an emphasis was a wholesome corrective. Many patients did seek psychiatric treatment because of their disproportionate sense of sin—because of "overdeveloped superegos" in psychiatric parlance. But now, one hundred years later, we seem to have learned only too well the lessons which early psychiatrists tried to teach, and the pendulum may have swung too far in the other direction.

During the past thirty or forty years many parents have feared that they will constrict their children's emotional and intellectual development and inhibit their freedom and creativity if they discipline them too much. And now many patients seek treatment because their underdeveloped conscience and sense of guilt has gotten them into trouble. Although they usually do not recognize the deficiency and present it as their primary problem, "too little superego" has led them to undisciplined or self-centered behavior, and they usually seek treatment in the groping awareness that the consequences of such behavior are social rejection and a sense of personal emptiness and restlessness. Confronted with such patients, psychiatrists are just beginning to recognize and emphasize that we must reassess our priorities, that a sense of sin may at times be quite a good thing.

Several case histories may further illustrate the nature of the problem which psychiatry and religion confront.

> Mr. Miller was admitted to a psychiatric unit because of overwhelming feelings of despondency. At sixty-four and in ill health, he felt he was going to die soon and that damnation was certain. He sat for hours musing over sins that he had committed over the years—ranging from occasionally failing to attend church because he wanted to go fishing to a premarital sexual experience which he had in his early twenties. His despair was so great that he was seriously contemplating suicide, certain that damnation was inevitable anyway. He refused to eat, lost twenty pounds, and slept only two or three hours a night, typically awakening after only a few hours of fitful

sleep to ruminate about his fallen nature and his multiple (but actually not very serious) sins.

Mr. Wilson came in initially with his wife for what was identified as a "marital problem." Both were in their early twenties and had been married for about a year, although they lived together for a year prior to their marriage. Mrs. Wilson was in her fifth month of pregnancy, and her husband felt the main problem was the stress which the pregnancy placed on them. She was often tired, was working fulltime to supplement the rather limited income he made as a trumpet player, and was no longer as quick to perform household chores or to respond sexually. She also described some mild depressive symptoms. In the course of therapy, it emerged that he was having an extramarital affair and that he tended to have a lifestyle characterized by taking advantage of others, emphasis on self-gratification, and a limited sense of responsibility toward his wife and child. The "marital problem" in this case was primarily due to his self-centered behavior, and eventually he (rather than his wife or the marriage) was identified as the primary focus for psychiatric treatment.

Obviously, Mr. Miller and Mr. Wilson have different kinds of problems. Mr. Miller suffered from a severe depressive illness, of which his preoccupation with sin and guilt was a symptom. His sense of guilt was developed to such an extent that it was disproportionate to his actual behavior, and therefore it was actually harming and handicapping him. One should emphasize that religion itself was not to blame for his illness, and ultimately the positive aspects of religion were used to help him as he recovered.

On the other hand, Mr. Wilson lacked an adequately developed conscience. His marriage was indeed failing, and in this case most of the responsibility for the failure fell on him, although he did not realize it initially. Therapy in his case involved helping him come to a realization of the destructive effects of his self-centered behavior and actually to experience a sense of guilt about his rather cavalier neglect of his wife's feelings and the pain he had caused her. He was then able to try to "make it right" to her and eventually achieved feelings of self-worth based on self-improvement that he had never experienced before. At one point in treatment he commented with surprise, "But I thought it was wrong to feel guilty." He gradually learned the distinction between pathological guilt, which he never experienced, and wholesome guilt, which he needed to experience more often. That is the major distinction upon which the problem of guilt in psychiatry depends.

Religion and Health: How Religion Enriches

Thus, a religious point of view, even one which places emphasis on sin and guilt, is not harmful for psychiatric patients. Some may overemphasize sin and develop pathological guilt, but that is due to illness rather than religion. Depressive symptoms tend to manifest themselves as pronounced guilt feelings in people with a religious background, while someone with a more secular point of view will simply develop other depressive symptoms. Most clergymen would agree that the severe pathological guilt of the depressive is a derangement of a potentially sound or healthy religious tenet, and both clergyman and psychiatrist would try to direct such patients toward the more comforting aspects of religion. Not only is a religious point of view not harmful; it may actually be extremely helpful.

For a psychiatric patient experiencing severe despair, suicide is always a significant risk. Although hard facts are not available, suicide seems to be increasing in incidence during the twentieth century, and this is probably related to the advancing tide of secularism. In earlier centuries suicide was always seen as an irrevocable sin leading to damnation, since it involved voluntary destruction of a life given by God and could not be propitiated or rectified since it led to death. For a religious person in the twentieth century, such reasoning can still serve as a deterrant. Even such a patient as Mr. Miller will usually respond to a line of reasoning which stresses the irrevocable quality of suicide—that he can commit suicide at any time if he really wishes to do so, but that his suffering may diminish in a few days or weeks and that deferring suicide until then is probably worthwhile since he has little to lose by waiting to see what the future holds but a great deal to lose if he commits suicide at once. Further, such patients can be reminded that God is merciful and loving, that no sin is too great to be forgiven, and great saints have experienced spiritual aridity similar to that from which they suffer.

Religion may also be helpful to other types of patients. For a patient such as Mr. Wilson, religion may help define a moral structure which will help him in building a superego or conscience. It is the superego which gives us a perspective by which to determine right from wrong, appropriateness from inappropriateness, value from valuelessness. My own experience leads me to prefer the teachings of Christianity. However, as a student of human behavior, I also know that each person resolves religious questions out of his own personal ethnic setting, language pattern, and social structure. And as a psychiatrist, I see how often we, as human beings, tend to turn our own descriptive confessions into prescriptive teachings which we then may use to denigrate the beliefs of others in order to enhance our own self-esteem. While I can speak confidently of my own experience with Christianity as valid and meaningful, if truth is one, then we must be open to the possibility that other experiences too may be valid and meaningful sources of truth. Some patients may find Judaeo-Christian tradition emotionally or intellectually unacceptable, for the time being at least, because they are in rebellion against many of the conventional values of Western society. Their right to inquire and reevaluate should be respected. Whatever intellectual position is most acceptable to them in building a moral framework and helping them to think in terms of a spiritual reality greater than themselves is of significant value in their process of personal growth.

Religion is potentially enriching or helpful in another sense as well. Not only does it provide a value system by which a person may live, but it also provides meaning and purpose for an individual's life. Life without a spiritual center runs a significant risk of being either shallow or empty. Perhaps a person who lives according to the pleasure principle, seeking gratification for himself alone as his primary goal in life, is as happy when all is going well for him as a person who lives according to spiritual principles. Perhaps not. Human beings being what they are—prone to rationalize and justify the pattern of behavior which they themselves pursue—a person who lives hedonistically is likely to affirm that he is living the good life, while a person who lives by spiritual values is likely to feel that his life is more fulfilling. But when things go badly, there is not much doubt who is happier, by either's testimony. The individual who values only material things or power can find no meaning for his life if he somehow loses them. The person who can confront loss or suffering with the help of religious values finds pain infinitely more bearable.

Existential Psychiatry and the Future

Providing new hope for an emphasis on the fourth dimension is a relatively new movement known as existential psychiatry. Leading figures in this movement have included Rollo May, Viktor Frankl, Karl Jaspers, and Medard Boss.

Although this school does not deny the contribution of the Freudian, behavioral, or medical points of view, it stresses the importance and value of spiritual and philosophical factors in human life.

A primary tenet of the existential school is an emphasis on choice and ethics. Looking back to the secular existentialist Jean Paul Sartre, an atheist but also a profound moralist, they assert with him that "existence precedes essence." Fundamentally, that statement means that our behavior determines what we are and what we become. The choices that we make in the process of existing determine the essence that we have. In Sartre's words, "we are our choices." The practical result of this point of view is that great responsibility is placed on the individual for the direction and shape which his life will take. Although he may come from a neurotogenic background, he *is* able to overcome it slowly through the manner of his existence. Each time he acts his personality takes on the moral quality of his act. Each time he performs a kindness, he becomes a kinder person. Each time he gives another person his faith and trust, he becomes a more trusting person. And, contrariwise, if he chooses to move in the direction of evil, he becomes the evil that he performs. Behavior, personality, and moral character are all interwoven.

A second tenet of the existential school is the emphasis on individuality. This is a corollary of the emphasis on individual moral responsibility. This tenet stresses that the clinician and scientist should focus their attention on the distinctive qualities of each individual's conscious experience rather than to try to fit him to the procrustean bed of a psychological framework such as Freudianism or behaviorism. This tenet is based on the teachings of a philosophical school known as phenomenonology, particularly well expressed by the psychiatrist and existential philosopher Karl Jaspers, which stresses that mental phenomena are best understood by attempting to understand the descriptions given of them by human beings. Therefore it is sometimes called the phenomenological approach. Practically speaking, this point of view leads to psychotherapy which focuses on the personal experience of each individual patient. *His* perception of his pains and concerns is the main focus of attention, and in therapy both therapist and patient attempt to understand his experience, its meaning, and ways to surmount his personal pain.

A final tenet of the existential school is the emphasis on man's search for meaning in his life. Viktor Frankl in particular has argued that Freud is wrong in defining the fundamental human drives as sex and aggression. He believes that the most fundamental drive is toward finding meaning and purpose. Man shares sex and aggression with the rest of the animal world, but man is distinguished from the animal world through his search for a spiritual center which has greater value and magnitude than his individual existence. Practically speaking, this means that many patients who seek treatment are in fact seeking help in finding a purpose to their lives. From Frankl's point of view, psychotherapy with this type of patient should be a logotherapy, a therapy which assists the patient in finding a logos or spiritual center. Rather than dwelling morbidly on his pain and personal suffering, the patient seeks to find a meaning for that suffering which will give his life a purpose or goal.

Although it cannot begin to resolve all the problems about how the mind works or how people can best be helped, the existential school has provided a wholesome corrective to the Freudian emphasis on man as a helpless victim of neurotic drives and the behavioral emphasis on man as a soulless being who can be mechanically manipulated by a system of rewards and punishments. Existential psychiatry is a relatively young and amorphous school in the process of evolving its points of view. As it continues to work toward defining its essences, we can all learn a great deal from it.

Suggested Further Reading

OF GENERAL INTEREST

Jones, E. *The Life and Works of Sigmund Freud*. Basic Books: New York, 1961.

Stone, I. *The Passions of the Mind*. Signet: New York, 1972.

Menninger, K. *Love Against Hate*. Harvest Books: New York, 1942.

Fromm, E. *The Art of Loving*. Bantam: New York, 1956.

Fromm, E. *The Heart of Man*. Harper and Row: New York, 1968.

Hastings, D. W. *A Doctor Speaks on Sexual Expression in Marriage*. Bantam: New York, 1966.

Laycock, S. R. *Family Living and Sex Education*. Mil-Mac Publications: Toronto, 1967.

BIOGRAPHICAL AND
AUTOBIOGRAPHICAL ACCOUNTS

Kaplan, B., ed., *The Inner World of Mental Illness*. Harper and Row: New York, 1964.

Beers, C. *A Mind That Found Itself*. Longmans, Green: New York, 1908.

Boisen, A. *Out of the Depths*. Harper and Row: New York, 1960.

Green, H. *I Never Promised You a Rose Garden*. Signet: New York, 1964.

Lindner, R. *The Fifty Minute Hour*. Bantam: New York, 1955.

TYPES OF ILLNESS

Schizophrenia: *Is There an Answer?* HEW Publications No. 73-0986, 1972 (Sold by Superintendent of Documents, U.S. Government Printing Office, Washington, D.C. 20402).

Cammer, L. *Up from Depression.* Simon and Shuster: New York, 1969.

Winokur, G., Clayton, P., and Reich, T. *Manic Depressive Illness.* C. V. Mosby: St. Louis, 1969.

Fenichel, O. *The Psychoanalytical Theory of Neurosis.* W. W. Norton: New York, 1945.

Veith, I. *Hysteria: The History of a Disease.* University of Chicago Press: Chicago and London, 1965.

Salzman, L. *The Obsessive Personality.* Science House: New York, 1968.

Alcohol and Alcoholism. PHS Publication No. 1640, 1969 (Sold by U.S. Government Printing Office, as above).

Manual on Alcoholism. American Medical Association, 1970 ($2.00, Sold by AMA, 535 North Dearborn St., Chicago, Ill.).

Drug Dependence: A Guide for Physicians. American Medical Association, 1969 ($1.00, Sold by AMA, as above).

CAUSES OF PSYCHIATRIC DISORDER

GENERAL

Million, T. *Theories of Psychopathology*. W. B. Saunders: Philadelphia and London, 1967.

MEDICAL MODEL

Himwich, H. E. *Biochemistry, Schizophrenias, and Affective Illnesses*. Williams and Wilkins: Baltimore, 1970.

BEHAVIORAL MODEL

Skinner, B. F. *Science and Human Behavior*. Free Press: New York, 1953.

PSYCHOANALYTIC MODEL

Freud, S. *A General Introduction to Psychoanalysis*. Permabooks: New York, 1924.

Erickson, E. *Childhood and Society*. W. W. Norton: New York, 1950.

TREATMENT METHODS

Hersher, L. *Four Psychotherapies.* Appleton, Century, Crofts: New York, 1970.

Brenner, C. *An Elementary Textbook of Psychoanalysis.* Doubleday Anchor: New York, 1957.

Hall, C. S. *A Primer of Freudian Psychology.* Mentor Books: New York, 1954.

Wolpe, J. *The Practice of Behavior Therapy.* Pergamon Press: New York, 1969.

Kalinowsky, L. B. and Hippius, H. *Pharmacological, Convulsive and Other Somatic Treatments in Psychiatry.* Grune and Stratton: New York, 1969.

Yalom, I. D. *The Theory and Practice of Group Psychotherapy.* Basic Books: New York, 1970.

Schutz, W. C. *Joy.* Grove Press: New York, 1969 (on T groups).

Satir, V. *Conjoint Family Therapy.* Science and Behavior Books: Palo Alto, Calif., 1967.

RELIGION AND PSYCHIATRY

Mowrer, O. H. *The Crisis in Psychiatry and Religion*. Van Nostrand: Princeton, N.J., 1961.

Frankl, V. E. *Man's Search for Meaning*. Washington Square Press: New York, 1963.

Szasz, T. S. *The Myth of Mental Illness*. Harper and Row: New York, 1961.

James, W. *The Varieties of Religious Experience*. Modern Library: New York, 1902.

Cole, W. G. *Sex in Christianity and Psychoanalysis*. Galaxy: New York, 1966.

Erikson, E. H. *Young Man Luther*. W. W. Norton: New York, 1958.